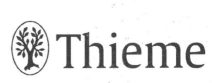

Lumbar Interbody Fusion

Pearls and Techniques

Editor-in-Chief

Satish Rudrappa, MCh (Neurosurgery), FASS (USA), FRCS (Glasgow)
Director,
Sakra Institute of Neurosciences,
Head,
Department of Spine Surgery,
Sakra World Hospital,
Bangalore, Karnataka, India

Editorial Board

Ramachandran Govindasamy, MS (Ortho), DNB (Ortho)
Department of Spine Surgery,
Sakra Institute of Neurosciences,
Bangalore, Karnataka, India

Veeramani Preethish-Kumar, MRCP (UK), MD-PhD (ICMR Fellow)
Department of Spine Surgery,
Sakra Institute of Neurosciences,
Bangalore, Karnataka, India

Thieme
Delhi • Stuttgart • New York • Rio de Janeiro

Publishing Director: Ritu Sharma
Development Editor: Dr Nidhi Srivastava
Director-Editorial Services: Rachna Sinha
Project Manager: Sambhavi Shah, Nidhi Chopra
Vice President, Sales and Marketing: Arun Kumar Majji
Managing Director & CEO: Ajit Kohli

Thieme Medical and Scientific Publishers Private Limited.
A - 12, Second Floor, Sector - 2, Noida - 201 301,
Uttar Pradesh, India, +911204556600
Email: customerservice@thieme.in
www.thieme.in

Cover design: Thieme Publishing Group
Typesetting by RECTO Graphics, India

Printed in India

5 4 3 2 1

ISBN: 978-93-88257-54-1
eISBN: 978-93-88257-55-8

Important note: Medicine is an ever-changing science undergoing continual development. Research and clinical experience are continually expanding our knowledge, in particular, our knowledge of proper treatment and drug therapy. Insofar as this book mentions any dosage or application, readers may rest assured that the authors, editors, and publishers have made every effort to ensure that such references are in accordance with **the state of knowledge at the time of production of the book.**

Nevertheless, this does not involve, imply, or express any guarantee or responsibility on the part of the publishers in respect to any dosage instructions and forms of applications stated in the book. **Every user is requested to examine carefully** the manufacturers' leaflets accompanying each drug and to check, if necessary, in consultation with a physician or specialist, whether the dosage schedules mentioned therein or the contraindications stated by the manufacturers differ from the statements made in the present book. Such examination is particularly important with drugs that are either rarely used or have been newly released in the market. Every dosage schedule or every form of application used is entirely at the user's own risk and responsibility. The authors and publishers request every user to report to the publishers any discrepancies or inaccuracies noticed. If errors in this work are found after publication, errata will be posted at www.thieme.com on the product description page.

Some of the product names, patents, and registered designs referred to in this book are in fact registered trademarks or proprietary names even though specific reference to this fact is not always made in the text. Therefore, the appearance of a name without designation as proprietary is not to be construed as a representation by the publisher that it is in the public domain.

Contents

Foreword

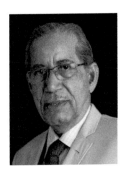

I am pleased to know that Dr. Satish Rudrappa, President of Neuro Spinal Surgeon's Association, has compiled a monograph on lumbar inter-body fusion (LIF) to be released on the occasion of 2019 Neuro Spinal Surgeon's Conference. It is pleasing to note that in this era of minimally invasive spinal surgeries, the editor-in-chief has chosen to compile the history, evolution, and recent developments in the field of LIF, which clearly indicates its enormous importance in the field.

The most important aspect in treating spinal disorders is the maintenance of sagittal balance as mentioned by the editor in his column. It is indeed the anchor for a good functioning spine.

The editor has taken pains to invite contributors from across the world to cover each and every aspect of the topic so that the monograph looks almost like a book in the archives. Right from the good old posterior LIF that I practiced and propagated, to the writing on minimally invasive surgery (MIS), and endoscopic transforaminal LIF, the editor has made humungous efforts to compile these methodically. The editor-in-chief has also vividly described the techniques of MIS which all aspiring young spinal surgeons will find educative.

Oblique or anterior techniques are re-emerging, especially in surgeries to treat deformities. But the general feeling that everything can be approached by posterior routes has kept these approaches dormant. However, the re-emergence of these techniques and their utilities have been well-described by the contributors who have written the chapters. For a person like me, these chapters hold extreme importance from the point of view of recent developments in LIF techniques.

In the current world, there is a big hue and cry over the implants being overused. The message from the chapter on "Implants and Biologics in Lumbar Interbody Fusion" should be perceived intelligently.

Dr. Satish Rudrappa is not only a hardworking and intelligent neuro spinal surgeon, but also highly research-oriented in the field of medicine. I am confident that this monograph will prove to be instructive and a useful bible for all the readers. I would also like to keep a personal copy in my library.

Dr. P. S. Ramani
Founder President, Neuro Spinal Surgeons Association, India

Note from the Editor-in-Chief

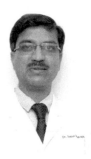

It is fascinating to see how lumbar spine surgery has evolved over centuries, from external manipulation to endoscopy guided minimally invasive surgical techniques in the recent decade. The most common pathology affecting the lumbar spine is degeneration.

There are different ways a surgeon thinks, in approaching a lumbar pathology. The ultimate aim for any surgeon in such a situation is to provide adequate decompression and reconstruct the spine to its normal anatomy as much as possible. Achieving sagittal balance of lumbosacral spine is the key for mobility in humans. Lumbar interbody fusion (LIF) is indispensable in restoring this balance in the diseased spine.

There are different approaches available for performing an LIF and the choice of surgery is influenced by multiple factors like patient's clinical presentation, X-ray, and MRI profile. Making the appropriate choice of surgery has a definite impact on postoperative long-term outcomes.

The purpose of this book is to discuss the advantages and shortcomings of each LIF procedure and the need to pick the right approach or a combination of approaches for the ultimate benefit of the patient. I sincerely believe and wish that the readers, especially spine surgeons, will benefit from this monograph.

Satish Rudrappa, MCh (Neurosurgery), FASS (USA), FRCS (Glasgow)

Contributors

Achal Gupta
Lilavati Hospital and Research Centre,
Mumbai, Maharashtra, India

Alvin Y. Chan
Department of Neurological Surgery,
University of California,
San Francisco, CA, USA

Andrew K. Chan
Department of Neurological Surgery,
University of California,
San Francisco, CA, USA

Apurva Prasad
Lilavati Hospital and Research Centre,
Mumbai, Maharashtra, India

**Arjun Dhawale, MS (Ortho), DNB (Ortho),
MRCS (Edinburgh)**
Consultant Spine Surgeon,
Department of Orthopedics and Spine Surgery,
Sir HN Reliance Foundation Hospital and
Research Center,
Mumbai, Maharashtra, India

Arvind Bhave, MS (Ortho), IPTM, EICOE,
Fellow Spinal Injuries (Japan)
Spine Surgeon and Spine Endoscopist,
Deenanath Mangeshkar Hospital,
Pune, Maharashtra, India

Dheeraj Masapu, MD, DM (Neuroanesthesia)
Associate Consultant,
Sakra Institute of Neurosciences,
Bengaluru, Karnataka, India

**J. K. B. C. Parthiban, MCh (Neurosurgery),
FNS (Japan)**
Senior Consultant,
Department of Neurosurgery,
Kovai Medical Center and Hospital,
Coimbatore, Tamil Nadu, India

Joshua J. Rivera
Department of Neurological Surgery,
University of California,
San Francisco, CA, USA

Justin M. Lee
Department of Neurological Surgery,
University of California,
San Francisco, CA, USA

Karl Janich, MD
Medical College of Wisconsin,
Milwaukee, WI, USA

**Komal Prasad Chandrachari, MS, DNB,
MCh (Neurosurgery), PGDHHM, PGDMLE, MNAMS**
Senior Consultant Neurosurgeon and Spinal Surgeon,
Narayana Hrudayalaya Institute of Neurosciences,
Mazumdar Shaw Medical Center, NH Health City,
Bengaluru, Karnataka, India

Kshitij Chaudhary, MS (Ortho), DNB (Ortho), FACS
Consultant Spine Surgeon,
Department of Orthopaedics and Spine Surgery,
Sir HN Reliance Foundation Hospital and
Research Center,
Mumbai, Maharashtra, India

Kumar Abhinav
Lilavati Hospital and Research Centre,
Mumbai, Maharashtra, India

Naresh K. Pagidimarry, MS
Barat Academy of Spine Endoscopy (BASE),
Hyderabad, India

Peng Yin
Department of Orthopaedics,
Beijing Chao-Yang Hospital, China Capital
Medical University,
Beijing, China

Praveen V. Mummaneni, MD
Department of Neurological Surgery,
Joan O'Reilly Endowed Chair,
Professor and Vice-Chairman
University of California,
San Francisco, USA

**P. S. Ramani, MBBS, MS, MSc Neurosurgery (UK),
DSc, FNAMS (National Academy)**
Senior Consultant
Neuro and Spinal Surgeon,
Lilavati Hospital and Research Centre,
Mumbai, Maharashtra, India

**Ramachandran Govindasamy, MS (Ortho),
DNB (Ortho)**
Spine Consultant,
Department of Spine Surgery,
Sakra Institute of Neurosciences,
Bangalore, Karnataka, India

Said G. Osman, MD, FRCS (Edinburgh) (Ortho)
Sky Spine Endoscopy Institute,
Frederick, MD, USA

Sajesh Menon, MS (Ortho), DNB (Ortho), MCh
Clinical Professor and Head,
Department of Neurosurgery,
Amrita Institute of Medical Science,
Kochi, Kerala, India

Satish Rudrappa, MCh (Neurosurgery), FASS (USA), FRCS (Glasgow)
Director, Sakra Institute of Neurosciences,
Head, Department of Spine Surgery,
Sakra World Hospital,
Bengaluru, Karnataka, India

S. N. Kurpad, MD-PhD
Sanford J Larson Professor and Chairman,
Department of Neurosurgery,
Medical College of Wisconsin,
Milwaukee, WI, USA

Sukumar Sura, MCh (Neurosurgery), FRCS (Edinburgh)
Department of Neurosurgery,
Yashoda Hospitals, Hyderabad, India

Sumeet Sasane
Lilavati Hospital and Research Centre,
Mumbai, Mumbai, Maharashtra, India

T. V. Ramakrishna, MS (Ortho), FISS & FISD (Japan)
Department of Neurosurgery,
Yashoda Hospitals, Hyderabad, India

Veeramani Preethish-Kumar, MRCP (UK), MD-PhD (ICMR Fellow)
Associate Consultant,
Academic and Research Head,
Sakra Institute of Neurosciences,
Bengaluru, Karnataka, India

Vivian P. Le
Department of Neurological Surgery,
University of California,
San Francisco, USA

Yaoshen Zhang
Department of Orthopaedics,
Beijing Chao-Yang Hospital, China Capital
Medical University,
Beijing, China

Yiqi Zhang
Department of Orthopaedics,
Beijing Chao-Yang Hospital, China Capital
Medical University,
Beijing, China

Yong Hai, MD-PhD
Professor, Department of Orthopaedics,
Beijing Chao-Yang Hospital,
China Capital Medical University,
Beijing, China

Yu Liang, MD
Professor, Deputy Chief,
Director, Spine Division,
Department of Orthopaedics,
Ruijin Hospital, School of Medicine,
JiaoTong University, Shanghai, China

Chapter 1
History of Lumbar Interbody Fusion

1 History of Lumbar Interbody Fusion

P. S. Ramani, Sumeet Sasane, Apurva Prasad, Achal Gupta, Kumar Abhinav

Introduction

History is very important and an integral component of any man-made technological advancement, especially in the field of medicine. The history of treatment for any spinal disease follows the same path as any other medical illness dating to the beginning of human history. Indian and Egyptian texts reveal descriptions of spinal instability as early as ca. 1550 BC. Hippocrates (460–377 BC), the Greek physician, may have been a pioneer in describing spinal conditions in a scientific manner, and many physicians followed his teachings.[1,2] Hence, it is evident that the concept of "spine correction and stabilization" existed for centuries, but the way to do so was not clear until the late 19th century (**Fig. 1.1**). Today, in the modern era, numerous surgical techniques are available for the stabilization of the spine. After reviewing from a historical perspective, it will be apparent how dependent we remain upon the work of those who came before us so that we can write further on any new advances. However, many times new discoveries are serendipitous.

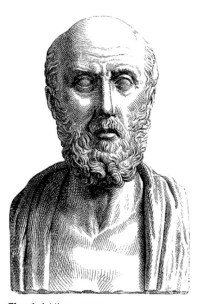

Fig. 1.1 Hippocrates.

Historical Background

The evolution of external spine-fixation devices was during the 15th and 16th century when physicians tried to understand the complex biomechanical mechanisms of the spine.[3,4] Later, the management paradigm shifted toward surgery because of the discovery of anesthesia and antisepsis in 1846 and 1867, respectively.[5] The first surgical attempt in spine was by Berthold Hadra,[6] a Prussia-based surgeon from Texas, in 1891. He attempted to stabilize an 8-month-old dislocated fracture of the sixth and seventh cervical vertebrae. He incised from occiput to first thoracic vertebra and tried to fuse the adjacent spinous processes using silver wires in a figure-of-8 fashion (**Fig. 1.2**). But he was modest enough to give the credit to Wilkins, who had successfully done a similar procedure before him in treating a dislocated fracture of the dorsolumbar region. There was a substantial rise in tuberculosis (TB) leading to a high prevalence of Pott's spine and spinal deformities in the 18th and 19th century. This leads to the discovery of internal stabilization of spine starting from cervical spine and gradually finding its way to the lumbar spine. Following Hadra, Chipault performed the same wiring technique for internal fixation of five Pott's spine cases by 1895.[7] In 1908, Fritz Lange[8] tied tin-plated steel rods to the spine with wires. However, he gave up on using steel due to corrosion issues.

The Concept of Spinal Fusion Using "On-Lay" Bone Graft

Fred Albee[9] and Russel Hibbs[10] from New York laid the scientific foundation for lumbar fusion through their technique of posterior on-lay bone grafting for patients with TB spine. They published their results independently in 1911. Later, surgeons adapted the same technique for the correction of scoliosis or spinal fractures.

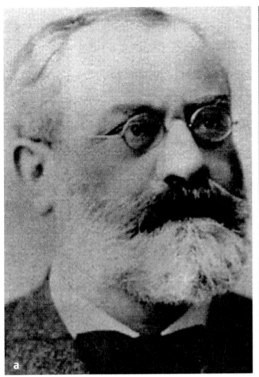 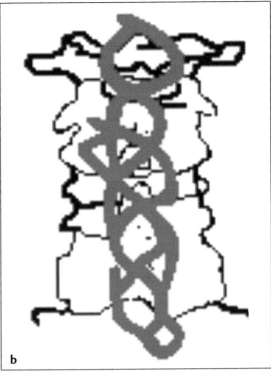

Fig. 1.2 Berthold Ernest Hadra **(a)**, a physician and surgeon from Prussia who revolutionized spinal surgical techniques and the figure-of-8 interspinous wiring **(b)**.

This technique was further elaborated by other surgeons adding iliac crest or tibial bone grafts. As a matter of interest, within a short period of time, Albee preceded Hibbs in using grafts. He compared the strength of bone grafting over internal metal splints and found high rates of failure of rods and wires due to direct absorption and bone atrophy.

Posterior approach gained popularity and small case series on spine instrumentations started coming up. Campbell in 1920 first described trisacral fusion through autografting from iliac crest to the transverse processes of L4/L5 vertebrae.[11] This is the first documented "lumbosacral fusion" technique, which laid the foundation for successive posterior spinal instrumentation techniques. However, nonunion due to corrosion of implants was a major concern. In 1933, Ghormley[12] used iliac crest grafts on the transverse processes for fusion and following this, it became the procedure of choice and gained popularity among contemporary surgeons.

In 1936, Venable and Stuck introduced Vitallium[13] (an alloy of cobalt, chromium, and molybdenum) that was inert and resistant to corrosion, overcoming the major issue with steel. In the late 1940s, King adapted Hibbs' technique by adding facet screw.[14–16] He was the first to use vertebral screw fixation and thereby immediately obtaining good rigid fixation, avoiding prolonged brace immobilization. But the short screws in the facets resulted in high incidence of pseudoarthrosis.[17] Despite several modifications to the technique, the incidence of pseudoarthrosis remained an ever-unsolvable problem in surgeries with on-lay bone grafting.

Evolution of "Interbody" Fusion Procedures of the Lumbar Spine

The Anterior Lumbar Interbody Fusion

The anterior approaches emerged in the 1930s (by Burns and Capener) mainly for treating spondylolisthesis. In 1933, Burns performed anterior fusion, through an anterior transperitoneal approach by left paramedian incision, drilling a hole in the fifth lumbar vertebra and filling it with autograft. This procedure had good postoperative outcome but the recovery was prolonged. This anterior approach claimed to have key advantages.[18,19] It provides a direct midline view of the disc space and efficient preparation, leading to high fusion rates. It also facilitates maximization of the implant size and surface area and, thereby, aggressive correction of lordosis and foraminal height. Nonetheless, Mobbs et al[20] reported approach-related complications such as retrograde ejaculation and visceral and vascular injury. Moreover, anterior lumbar interbody fusion (ALIF) is not suitable at L2–L4 vertebral level (retroperitoneal retraction and risk of superior mesenteric artery thrombosis).

Posterior Lumbar Interbody Fusion

Since anterior approaches were associated with significant morbidity and prolonged recovery time, Briggs and Milligan in 1944 revolutionized fusion surgeries and described a novel technique, combining a posterior approach with interbody fusion technique. It involved wide laminectomy, facetectomy, discectomy, and usage of a round bone peg for stability. This principle was later adapted by Cloward[21] and he described the first posterior lumbar interbody fusion (PLIF) procedure with few modifications. He used multiple small tricortical grafts from the posterior iliac crest and allografts from cadaver, thus further improving fusion rates up to 85%.[21] However, this was not gaining popularity, as it was very difficult and not every surgeon could achieve his expertise. Several surgeons adapted their own techniques to make PLIF simpler and more attractive, so that maximum number of surgeons can use it.

Lin from Philadelphia was one of the spinal surgeons who successfully advocated PLIF using only cancellous bone from the posterior iliac crest.[22] He described the principle of "Unipour Concept." His concepts were also based on "Flagpole concept" as described by a biomechanical engineer named Evans.[23] It states that a flagpole should be rooted to the ground by three wires so that it can remain stable. In a spine scenario, the three wires are anterior longitudinal ligament, facet joints laterally, and the interspinous and supraspinous ligaments. The lumbar interbody fusion (LIF) represents the flagpole here. However, there were shortcomings with Lin's construct as it was too soft and caused early settlement with foraminal stenosis. Despite all these modifications, standalone posterior interbody fusion fell out of favor due to technical difficulties, potential serious complications, and low fusion rates.

Ramani's construct contains a mixture of cancellous portion of bone (auto and allo) to make a 5-mm layer at the base and at the sides.[24] He added two tricortical bone graft from his own bone bank in the center and two bicortical bone graft from the posterior iliac crest, which improved the fusion rates (**Fig. 1.3**).

Understanding Spinal Biomechanics—Emergence of the Pedicle Screw

Up till this stage, following any spinal fusion procedure, the patients had to be immobilized for a prolonged period; at least 6 weeks depending on the extent of instability. They will be cautiously mobilized with rigid lumbar brace, with or without hip lock, and will be allowed to sit up only after another 2 weeks. After spending several months postoperatively, walking would be initiated but by then, most of the patients will lose the zeal to work anymore.

Boucher described placing screws in the pedicle in 1959, but it was Roy Camille from France in 1970 who described sagittal screw placement across three columns: from articular process through the pedicle into the body and combined them with a plate construct.[16] Harrington combined pedicle screws with his rod system, which was originally developed for treating scoliosis (**Fig. 1.4**). He felt that standalone spinal instrumentation without fusion often resulted in implant failure owing to a race between development of fusion and failing implant material. The insight that instrumentation and bone grafting should be combined was a major step ahead in spine surgery.[25,26]

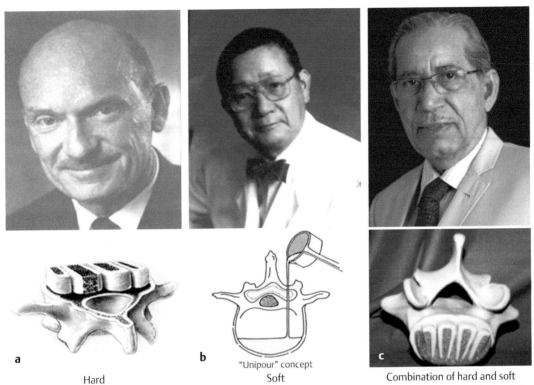

Fig. 1.3 (a–c) The three different constructs for posterior lumbar interbody fusion (lower panels) and the contributors: **(a)** Cloward, **(b)** Lin, and **(c)** Ramani (upper panels). The last construct has 5-mm thickness bone chips at the bottom and, at the sides, two central tricortical allografts, and two lateral bicortical autografts.

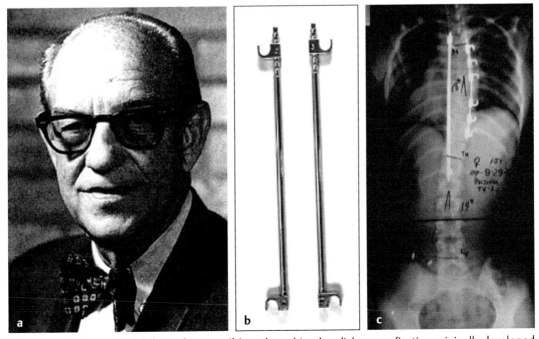

Fig. 1.4 Paul Harrington **(a)**, his rod system **(b)**, and combined pedicle screw fixation originally developed for treating scoliosis **(c)**.

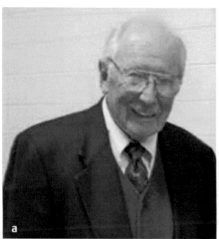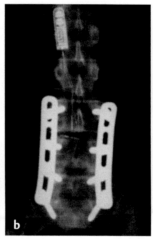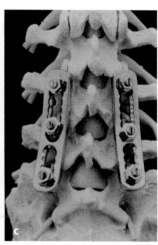

Fig. 1.5 Arthur Steffee (a) and his pedicle screw system/variable screw placement (VSP) plate (b and c).

In 1988, an orthopaedic surgeon named Steffee combined pedicle screw and/or variable screw placement plate along with LIF to restore load sharing through the anterior column. This led to increased stability and higher fusion rates[27] (Fig. 1.5) with early postoperative mobilization and significant reduction in hospital stay.

Transforaminal Lumbar Interbody Fusion

Harms and Rolinger[28,29] introduced transforaminal lumbar interbody fusion (TLIF) in 1998 and they did transforaminal approach, inserting a single kidney-shaped cage to achieve interbody fusion. The approach is unilateral through the intervertebral foramen and does not involve the canal, preventing postoperative fibrosis. Compared with PLIF, it is less destructive, and therefore considered to be safer than previous techniques. From 1970 to 1980s, using bone alone for inter-body fusion was a concern as it created settlement of disc space over a long period of time. Metallic cages were then introduced starting with Bagby[30] who inserted a horse shoe-shaped metallic cage for cervical interbody fusion. This trend was followed for different surgeries, and surgeons invented different types of cages for LIF. They were initially manufactured with stainless steel, which interfered with MRIs. To solve this problem, in 1989, titanium metal was used instead of stainless steel.[31,32] Till now, it has stood the test of time

and usage of titanium metal pedicle screws and cages is still in practice. Although MRI is possible with this metal, it still produces artifacts but, comparatively, much lesser than the earlier materials. It can be overcome by using high-resolution MRI to a certain extent as visualization of soft tissue is still impaired.

Another material named polyether ethyl ketone (PEEK) was introduced by Williams in 1987.[33] It has enough strength, but it is not too rigid and hence was not in routine use, especially in lumbar fusion surgeries. However, the first PEEK cage[34,35] was introduced only in 1999 as they found it to be wear, fatigue resistant, and radiolucent, and then surgeons started using it more commonly in cervical spine surgeries and less commonly in lumbar spine.

Lumbar Lateral Interbody Fusion/Extreme Lateral Interbody Fusion/Direct Lateral Interbody Fusion

Okuda et al, found a 25% complication rate with PLIF and the most common intraoperative complication was dural tear, with the most serious complication being severe postoperative neurological deficits.[36] Surgical time and blood loss have been implicated in higher rates especially in elderly causing morbidity. Hence, there was a need for a procedure with less perioperative morbidity, less invasiveness, using smaller portals, and minimizing soft tissue damage. Lateral lumbar interbody fusion was first introduced by Pimenta et al in 2001, which allows for anterior vertebral column access using only two small incisions laterally. It prevents many complications of either an anterior approach, including vascular and visceral injury, or those of a posterior approach—paraspinal muscle denervation, dural tear, and neurological injury from dural retraction.

Oblique Lumbar Interbody Fusion

While direct lateral interbody fusion (DLIF) was advocated as a minimally invasive alternative to ALIF, it involves access to the interbody space through a transpsoas approach and possible injury to the psoas and lumbar plexus.[37] Moreover, accessing the L5-S1 space is difficult owing to interference by the iliac crest.

In 1997 Michael Meyer described a prepsoas approach accessing the disc space obliquely—the oblique LIF. It does not involve dissection of the psoas muscle, thus minimizing the risk of lumbar plexus injury and eliminating the need for neural monitoring during surgery. He also demonstrated the procedure at L5-S1 level and concluded that it can be adapted as a minimally invasive approach for access of all vertebral levels from L2 to S1.[38]

Minimally Invasive Spine: Transforaminal Lumbar Interbody Fusion

The tubular retractor spine systems, which have proved to be the workhorse of minimally invasive spine surgery (MISS) in current date, were introduced by Kevin Foley and his colleagues in 1994. Combining its application with percutaneous pedicle screw insertion, the technique of minimally invasive surgery (MIS)-TLIF was described in 2005.[39] MIS-TLIF retains all the advantages of TLIF, while minimizing the iatrogenic muscle injury (preserves the natural posterior tension band) and retraction-associated complications of an open procedure, described

as "fusion disease" by Kawaguchi et al.[40] MIS-TLIF significantly reduces the short-term morbidity of any open procedure.

Endoscopic: Transforaminal Lumbar Interbody Fusion

In the last decade, MIS-TLIF has gained wide spread popularity; however, the technique still requires an open incision of the muscles for tube placement. In parallel, endoscopic technologies in several other surgical fields were flourishing, which led to the emergence of endoscopic transforaminal techniques with the same goal of achieving minimal blood loss as MIS-TLIF. The different techniques of endo-TLIF include percutaneous endoscopy, biportal, and microendoscopy.[41] Endo-TLIF is an emerging technique in the field of MISS with promising benefits of minimal tissue damage and low rate of complications. However, the published studies using Endo-TLIF are less and the current level of evidence for clinical safety and effectiveness is low.

Conclusion

LIF surgeries have been practiced more frequently in the last decade than before, with significant refinement in the surgical techniques. There is more importance given to minimize tissue handling and destruction, which is indirectly driving the evolution of newer procedures. Unfortunately, with the evolution of newer technologies, newer challenges are on the rise resulting in increased burden on the health cost. To overcome this, there is a need to maintain management plans in the best interest of the patient. Despite the earlier surgeries being destructive in nature, those efforts have taught us to understand the "spinal biomechanics" better and paved the way for revolutionizing the surgical management strategies. Authors are always indebted to the contribution of the past people and hope with anticipation that many new techniques are in the process of evolution. The ultimate aim of any advancement is augmenting the functional status of the patient and also minimizing the complications as far as possible.

References

1. Hughes JT. The Edwin Smith Surgical Papyrus: an analysis of the first case reports of spinal cord injuries. Paraplegia 1988;26(2):71–82
2. Naderi S, Andalkar N, Benzel EC. History of spine biomechanics: part I—the pre-Greco-Roman, Greco-Roman, and medieval roots of spine biomechanics. Neurosurgery 2007;60(2):382–390, discussion 390–391
3. Sari H, Misirlioglu TO, Akarirmak U, Hussain S, Kecebas HD. The historical development and proof of lumbar traction used in physical therapy. J Pharm Pharmacol 2014;2:87–94
4. Silver JR. History of the Treatment of Spinal Injuries. New York, NY: Springer; 2003
5. Robinson DH, Toledo AH. Historical development of modern anesthesia. J Invest Surg 2012;25(3):141–149
6. Hadra BE. Wiring of the spinous processes in Pott's disease. Trans Am Orthop Assoc 1981;4:206
7. Chipault A. Travaux De Neurologie Chirurgicale. Paris: L. Battaille; 1986
8. Lange F. Support of the spondylotic spine by means of buried steel bars attached to the vertebrae. Am J Orthop Surg (Phila Pa) 1910;8:344
9. Albee FH. Transplantation of a portion of the tibia into spine for Pott's disease. JAMA 1911;57:885
10. Hibbs RH. An operation for progressive spinal deformities. NY J Med 1911;93:1013
11. Campbell W. An operation for extra-articular fusion of sacroiliac joint. Surg Gynecol Obstet 1939;45:218–219
12. Ghormley RK. Low back pain with special reference to the articular facets with present attention of an operative procedure. JAMA 1933;101:1773
13. Venable CS, Stuck WG. Three years' experience with vitallium in bone surgery. Ann Surg 1941;114(2):309–315
14. King D. Internal fixation for lumbosacral fusion. J Bone Joint Surg Am 1948;30A(3):560–565
15. Mostofi SB. Who's Who in Orthopedics. London: Springer International Publishing; 2005
16. Kabins MB, Weinstein JN. The history of vertebral screw and pedicle screw fixation. Iowa Orthop J 1991;11:127–136
17. Thompson WAL, Ralston EL. Pseudarthrosis following spine fusion. J Bone Joint Surg Am 1949;31A(2):400–405
18. Hsieh PC, Koski TR, O'Shaughnessy BA, et al. Anterior lumbar interbody fusion in comparison with transforaminal lumbar interbody fusion: implications for the restoration of foraminal height, local disc angle, lumbar lordosis, and sagittal balance. J Neurosurg Spine 2007;7(4):379–386
19. Phan K, Thayaparan GK, Mobbs RJ. Anterior lumbar interbody fusion versus transforaminal lumbar interbody fusion—systematic review and meta-analysis. Br J Neurosurg 2015;29(5):705–711
20. Mobbs RJ, Phan K, Daly D, Rao PJ, Lennox A. Approach-related complications of anterior lumbar interbody fusion: results of a combined spine and vascular surgical team. Global Spine J 2016;6(2):147–154
21. Cloward RB. The treatment of ruptured lumbar intervertebral discs by vertebral body fusion. I. Indications, operative technique, after care. J Neurosurg 1953;10(2):154–168
22. Lin PM, Cautilli RA, Joyce MF. Posterior lumbar interbody fusion. Clin Orthop Relat Res 1983;(180):154–168
23. Evans JH. Biomechanics of lumbar fusion. Clin Orthop Relat Res 1985;(193):38–46
24. Ramani PS. Posterior lumbar interbody fusion combined auto- and allograft technique. In: Yonenobu K, Ono K, Takemitsu Y, eds. Lumbar Fusion and Stabilization. Tokyo: Springer; 1993
25. Harrington PR, Dickson JH. Spinal instrumentation in the treatment of severe progressive spondylolisthesis. Clin Orthop Relat Res 1976;(117):157–163
26. Harrington PR, Tullos HS. Reduction of severe spondylolisthesis in children. South Med J 1969;62(1):1–7
27. Suk SI, Lee CK, Kim WJ, Lee JH, Cho KJ, Kim HG. Adding posterior lumbar interbody fusion to pedicle screw fixation and posterolateral fusion after decompression in spondylolytic spondylolisthesis. Spine 1997;22(2):210–219, discussion 219–220
28. Harms JG, Jeszenszky D. Die posteriore, lumbale, interkorporelle Fusion in unilateraler transforaminaler Technik. Oper Orthop Traumatol 1998;10(2):90–102
29. Harms J, Rolinger H. A one-stager procedure in operative treatment of spondylolistheses: dorsal traction-reposition and anterior fusion (author's transl) [in German]. Z Orthop Ihre Grenzgeb 1982;120(3):343–347
30. Bagby GW. Arthrodesis by the distraction-compression method using a stainless steel implant. Orthopedics 1988;11(6):931–934
31. Kuslich SD, Ulstrom CL, Griffith SL, Ahern JW, Dowdle JD. The Bagby and Kuslich method of lumbar interbody fusion. History, techniques, and 2-year follow-up results of a United States prospective, multicenter trial. Spine 1998;23(11):1267–1278, discussion 1279
32. Ray CD. Threaded titanium cages for lumbar interbody fusions. Spine 1997;22(6):667–679, discussion 679–680

33. William D, Mc Namara A, Turner R. Potential of polyether ether ketone (PEEK) and carbon fiber reinforced peek in medical applications. J Mater Sci Lett 1987;18:267–272

34. Brantigan JW, Steffee AD, Lewis ML, Quinn LM, Persenaire JM. Lumbar interbody fusion using the Brantigan I/F cage for posterior lumbar interbody fusion and the variable pedicle screw placement system: two-year results from a Food and Drug Administration investigational device exemption clinical trial. Spine 2000;25(11):1437–1446

35. Kurtz SM, Devine JN. PEEK biomaterials in trauma, orthopedic, and spinal implants. Biomaterials 2007;28(32):4845–4869

36. Okuda S, Oda T, Miyauchi A, et al. Lamina horizontalization and facet tropism as the risk factors for adjacent segment degeneration after PLIF. Spine 2008;33(25):2754–2758

37. Salzmann SN, Shue J, Hughes AP. Lateral lumbar interbody fusion-outcomes and complications. Curr Rev Musculoskelet Med 2017;10(4):539–546

38. Mayer HM. A new microsurgical technique for minimally invasive anterior lumbar interbody fusion. Spine 1997;22(6):691–699, discussion 700

39. Schwender JD, Holly LT, Rouben DP, Foley KT. Minimally invasive transforaminal lumbar interbody fusion (TLIF): technical feasibility and initial results. J Spinal Disord Tech 2005;18(Suppl):S1–S6

40. Kawaguchi Y, Matsui H, Tsuji H. Back muscle injury after posterior lumbar spine surgery. A histologic and enzymatic analysis. Spine 1996;21(8):941–944

41. Ahn Y, Youn MS, Heo DH. Endoscopic transforaminal lumbar interbody fusion: a comprehensive review. Expert Rev Med Devices 2019;16(5):373–380

Chapter 2
Indications for Lumbar Interbody Fusion

2 Indications for Lumbar Interbody Fusion

Satish Rudrappa, Ramachandran Govindasamy,
Veeramani Preethish-Kumar

Introduction

Lumbar interbody fusion (LIF) is an established treatment for numerous lumbar spine disorders, and the technique involves fusion of one lumbar vertebra with another for correcting an unstable segment. This procedure helps in the decompression of the neural elements, restoration of disc height, and lumbar lordosis achieved by placing an intervertebral cage in the disc space. Several approaches exist for performing an LIF surgery, which are broadly classified as anterior or posterior procedures based on the direction toward the transverse process[1] (**Fig. 2.1**). Anterior lumbar interbody fusion (ALIF), anterior to psoas/oblique lumbar interbody fusion (ATP/OLIF), and transpsoas/lateral lumbar interbody fusion (LLIF) are the anterior subtypes in which the access to disc and cage placement is anterior to the transverse process through the retroperitoneal corridor. Posterior lumbar interbody fusion (PLIF) and transforaminal lumbar interbody fusion (TLIF) approaches involve disc preparation and cage insertion from the posterior end through the neural element corridor. Though there are several other approaches available for performing an LIF surgery, the above-described methods are common in practice and they share common indications. However, there are some advantages/disadvantages of one procedure over another that have been substantially proven by various authors. Till date, there has been no definite class I evidence to prove the efficacy of one method over another in terms of the clinical outcomes and fusion rates.[2] In this chapter, the various

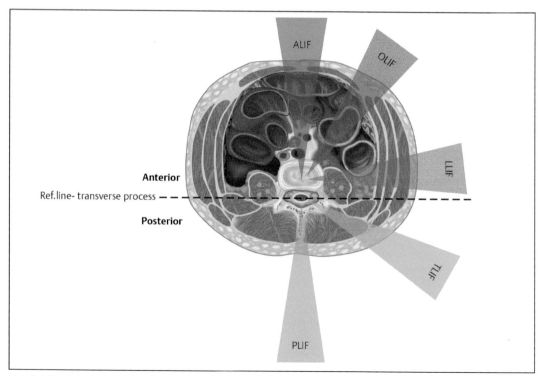

Fig. 2.1 Various types of lumbar interbody fusion.

indications of LIF and the advantages/disadvantages of the different approaches with respect to indications will be addressed.

Indications

The most common indication for spinal interbody fusion is "degeneration"[3] in which the common pathology is spondylolisthesis, where one vertebra translates over the adjacent vertebra resulting in back pain and neurological deterioration. The other pathologies and indications include spondylolysis, degenerative disc disease, disc prolapse, scoliosis, adjacent segment degeneration, postlaminectomy instability, pseudoarthrosis, spondylodiscitis, etc.[4] (**Table 2.1**).

The choice of interbody fusion in degeneration is usually decided by the following factors (**Box 2.1**).

Degenerative Low-Grade Spondylolisthesis

This condition is noticed predominantly in the seventh decade and especially in females. The listhesis usually occurs at L4–5 vertebral level where the upper vertebra translates over the other as a result of facetal degeneration. The neural element compression is secondary to a combination of multiple factors like ligamental flavum hypertrophy, facetal hypertrophy, disc prolapse, and reduced intervertebral height.[5]

The surgery for degenerative lumbar spondylolisthesis has evolved over a period of years from noninstrumented decompression and intertransverse fusion to minimally invasive surgery (MIS), which includes MIS-TLIF, MIS-LLIF, and MIS-OLIF. The choice of surgery is based on various factors; however, in general anterior/lateral procedures are recommended in patients with significantly reduced intervertebral height and minimum to moderate spinal canal stenosis (**Fig. 2.2**).[6] The posterior procedures have the advantage of 360-degree access to the spinal segment compared with the anterior procedures. PLIF is preferred in cases with significant central canal stenosis (ligamentum hypertrophy and claudication) but with a significant risk of dural and nerve root injuries[7] (**Fig. 2.3**). The transforaminal lumbar interbody fusion (TLIF) is of great value in case of lateral recess stenosis (facetal hypertrophy and radiculopathy) with a lesser risk of dural injuries[8] (**Fig. 2.4**). The ALIF procedure gives the maximum correction of lordosis among all the anterior methods.[9] LLIF, similar to ALIF, is found to have better listhesis reduction because of the ligamentotactic effect of larger profile cage and good mechanical stability.[10] Although there are various methods, several studies indicate that there is no significant difference in fusion rates,

Box 2.1 Factors influencing interbody fusion in degenerative lumbar disease

- Type and grade of spondylolisthesis
- Laterality of lateral recess and foraminal stenosis (facetal hypertrophy)
- Degree of central stenosis (ligamentum flavum hypertrophy)
- Coronal and sagittal imbalance
- Previous surgeries with/without interbody cages

Table 2.1 Surgical options based on indications

Pathological Indications	Type of LIF	Reason
Degenerative low-grade spondylolisthesis	PLIF/TLIF	Central canal stenosis/lateral recess stenosis
Degenerative adult spinal deformities—scoliosis and flat back	ALIF/OLIF/DLIF	Larger cage—better sagittal correction
High-grade spondylolisthesis	PLIF	Monosegmental/multisegmental safe
Degenerative disc diseases—back pain	ALIF	Muscle sparing approach
Spondylodiscitis	PLIF/TLIF	Safe procedure with neural decompression
Pseudoarthrosis	Circumferential	Based on previous surgery

Abbreviations: ALIF, anterior lumbar interbody fusion; DLIF, direct lumbar interbody fusion; OLIF, oblique lumbar interbody fusion; PLIF, posterior lumbar interbody fusion; TLIF, transforaminal lumbar interbody fusion.

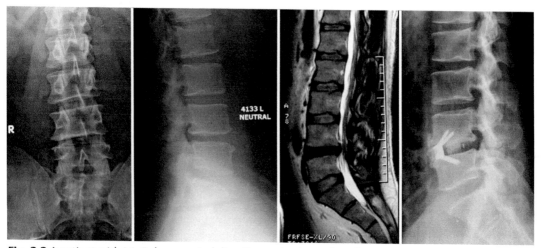

Fig. 2.2 A patient with L4–5 degenerated disc disease having reduced intervertebral disc height and mild canal stenosis treated by anterior lumbar interbody fusion.

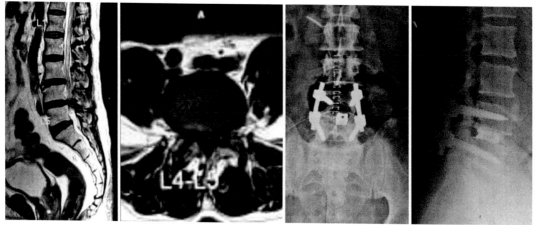

Fig. 2.3 A case of significant central lumbar canal stenosis treated by posterior lumbar interbody fusion.

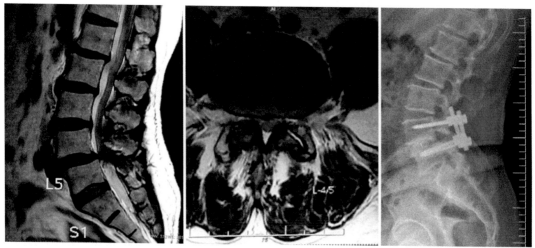

Fig. 2.4 A case of lateral recess stenosis with right radiculopathy treated by transforaminal lumbar interbody fusion.

but a definite difference in the rates of complication, for example, vascular injuries are high in ALIF and dural tears are high in PLIF.

With recent advancement and better understanding of MIS techniques, there has been a reduction in the rate of complications like prolonged time, radiculitis, dural injury, etc., with shorter hospital stay, lesser blood loss, and better alleviation of pain.[11] Though the cost of MIS implants is higher than open techniques, the overall cost of the procedure is almost identical in both the groups, as shown by some studies.[12,13] For a single-level degenerative spondylolisthesis with normal sagittal and coronal parameters, authors recommend posterior MIS or open TLIF/ PLIF based on the surgeon's expertise.

Adult Spinal Deformity (Degenerative Scoliosis and Flat Back)

With advancing age, degenerative changes of the disc, facets, and additional osteoporosis result in adult spinal deformity (ASD) both in coronal and sagittal plane. The sagittal deformity varies from flat back to kyphosis that will end up producing back pain, loss of posture, and horizontal field of vision, leading to significant disability. De novo scoliosis, a coronal deformity develops as a result of asymmetrical facet and disc changes and might result in neural compromise, especially on the concave side of the deformity.

Pseudoarthrosis, adjacent level fractures with kyphosis, adjacent segment degeneration, leading to instability and canal stenosis, are reported frequently in patients with preoperative sagittal and coronal imbalance. The parameters affecting the spinal balance have to be carefully considered in treating such patients.[14] Anterior procedures like ALIF, LLIF, or OLIF are better than posterior procedures in terms of lesser blood loss, shorter operative time, direct visualization of disc, better disc clearance, and larger disc space distraction.[15,16] The placement of larger cage in these procedures at anterior load-bearing region helps in restoring lumbar lordosis, with better coronal and sagittal balance and a lesser extent of instrumentation (**Fig. 2.5**). The anterior procedures are usually supplemented with posterior procedures like pedicle screw instrumentation to achieve a good spinal decompression. Crandall and Revella in their prospective nonrandomized study of anterior lumbar interbody fusion with posterior instrumentation of 20 patients had better fusion rates (80%) with improvement in Oswestry Disability Index and visual analogue scale scores similar to other studies.[17,18]

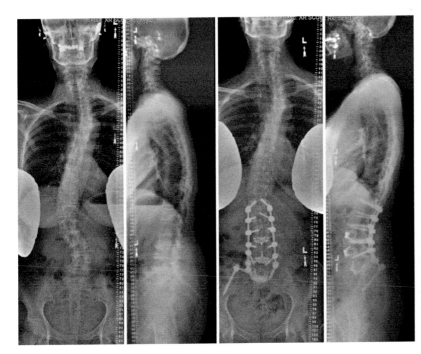

Fig. 2.5 Whole spine standing radiograph of a patient with adult spinal deformity treated by anterior lumbar interbody fusion and posterior spinal fusion.

The complexity in ASD is further worsened by factors like advanced age, co-morbidities, extensive blood loss, surgical site infections, and osteoporosis. The development of MIS techniques like OLIF/direct lumbar interbody fusion (DLIF)/percutaneous stabilization has reduced these complications to 12.1% in moribund elderly patients having ASDs.[19] Minimally invasive deformity surgery algorithm has been created by some authors based on sagittal parameters to guide for the decision making of an appropriate procedure, that is, MIS/open LIF.[20] Though the surgical procedures are complicated, these are very rewarding and often life changing. Authors recommend posterior spinal instrumentation with or without decompression and anterior LIF techniques in deformities of larger magnitude.

High-Grade Spondylolisthesis

The high-grade spondylolisthesis is characterized by Meyerding slip of more than 50% (Meyerding grade III, IV, V) and is usually dysplastic in etiology. The characteristics of dysplasia are trapezoidal L5, small L5 pedicles, sacral doming, elongated/broken pars, spina bifida, and dysplastic/aplastic facets. Conventionally, these slips were managed with in situ posterolateral fusion, or fibular strut grafts, or transdiscal screws, etc., in view of neurological damage expected to happen during reduction, but are reported with higher rates of nonunion. On the contrary, listhesis reduction and interbody fusion had higher fusion rates because of larger fusion surface, proper sagittal balance, and the grafts being placed at compression side.

In open posterior reduction and interbody fusions, the decompression of L5 nerve roots, adequate placement of L2/L3 or L4 screws for distraction if required, L5 screws for reduction, L5–S1 complete discectomy from bilateral sides, sacral osteotomy, and interbody fusion with cages are crucial steps. There are long-term studies of more than 10 years that demonstrate fusion and adequate sagittal balance, with no loss of reduction in "posterior only" procedures.[21] Though MIS procedures are highly demanding, it has been demonstrated to be safe and efficacious only in listhesis of grades II and III and not for grades IV and V.[22]

ALIF can reduce the translatory slip, maintain height, and thus can decompress the exiting nerve root in listhesis.[23] The stabilization can be done through standalone fixation with integral screws of the interbody cage, anterior plate fixation, or percutaneous screw fixation from the posterior aspect. Authors recommend fusion from L4–S1 with posterior interbody fusion (TLIF/PLIF) at L5–S1 for high-grade spondylolisthesis and ALIF/LLIF might not be the ideal choice as it is difficult to correct from anterior access.

Degenerative Disc Disease Related to Back Pain

The indication for fusion over conservative therapy in degenerative disc disease-related back pain is beyond the scope of this book, and in cases where it is indicated, ALIF is marginally better than other procedures owing to its muscle (paraspinal and psoas) sparing approach and better clearance of disc with removal of pain generators.[23] In degenerative disc disease (DDD), the potential pain generator is secondary to neoinnervation (neovascularization, neuronal penetration with unmyelinated nerve fibers, and the growth of Schwann cells). This subset of patients with radiculopathy will also benefit from anterior surgery as it indirectly decompresses the nerve by restoring the intervertebral disc height and thereby the foraminal height.

Pseudoarthrosis

Pseudoarthrosis is a failure in fusion of one vertebrae over another, usually postsurgery and requires revision surgeries in case of failed conservative treatment. The diagnosis of this condition might be evident in case of implant failures but may be a "diagnosis of exclusion" in some cases where the CT scans/stress films are equivocal. The revision surgery should address the technical errors, biomechanical errors with better graft materials, and should enhance the biological environment. It remains logical to go from an anterior in case of failed posterior arthrodesis, as approaching once again from the posterior might end up in higher chances of dural injuries and more morbidities. The vice versa may also hold true secondary to higher chances of vascular and visceral injuries, but there is no clear consensus regarding the same. The ALIF procedure has better fusion rates because of larger surface area, good vascularity from end plates, and compression loading of grafts.[24] The selection of procedure should be based on case to case. For example, removal of OLIF cage/ALIF cage is not possible from a posterior approach.

But in any procedure, correction of the biomechanical error, freshening the surfaces to enhance the biological environment, and usage of better bone graft materials are mandatory for achieving fusion (**Fig. 2.6**). Authors recommend a combined anteroposterior procedure for patients with pseudoarthrosis.

Spondylodiscitis

Spondylodiscitis is the infection of disc and end plates which can be tubercular, pyogenic, fungal, etc., and occurs secondary to hematogenous, direct, or iatrogenic spread. The most common method of treatment is conservative antibiotic therapy based on the organism. Surgery is recommended only in cases of instability, failure to respond with antibiotic therapy, neurological deficits, epidural abscess, deformities, and extensive destruction of the vertebrae >50% (**Fig. 2.7**). The aim of the treatment is to radically debride the disc material and achieve healing/fusion of the motion segment. Lin et al achieved satisfactory results in 22 patients of pyogenic spondylodiscitis treated by miniopen anterior debridement and interbody fusion with posterior percutaneous lumbar pedicle screws with less blood loss and acceptable postoperative complications.[25] Similar results were also obtained in extreme lateral lumbar interbody fusion (XLIF) procedures done for 27 pyogenic spondylodiscitis by Senthil et al with early recovery. The proponents of posterior procedure mention that anterior procedures in such chronic cases of spondylodiscitis might end up in complications owing to fibrosis with loss of

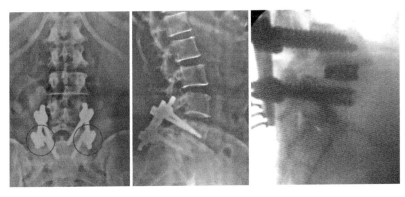

Fig. 2.6 Radiographs demonstrating pseudoarthrosis with implant failure for a high-grade L5–S1 spondylolisthesis.

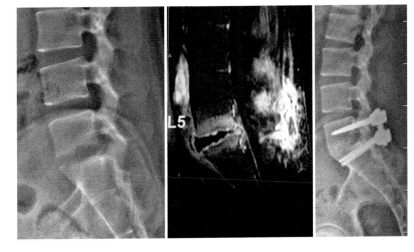

Fig. 2.7 A case of iatrogenic pyogenic spondylodiscitis treated by posterior lumbar interbody fusion using autologous bone grafts.

planes. Meng-Lin lu et al treated 30 spondylodiscitis of various organisms (MRSA [methicillin-resistant Staphylococcus aureus]-7, TB-3), by posterior TLIF and iliac bone grafts. All cases had healed infection, with 82.1% having a solid bone union, 10.7% inadequate union, and 7.2% of cases had nonunion. In most of the studies, the grafts are used as standalone in pyogenic spondylodiscitis without cages due to the risk of biofilm formation, but Shetty et al reported the safety of using metallic cages in 17 out of 27 pyogenic spondylodiscitis with no cage migration/loosening/pseudoarthrosis along with adequate clearance of infection and union.[26]

Preoperative Evaluation

In the quest for a proper clinical outcome, careful selection of the patient is the foremost requirement. For example, in a case of chronic low back pain in patients secondary to DDD, conservative measures including psychosomatic therapy have to be tried first and the pain generator has to be confirmed with discography. Further preoperative evaluation is a must in deciding the type of surgical procedure that will most suit the patient for satisfactory outcomes and limiting factors of each procedure have to be analyzed according to the levels of fusion (**Table 2.2**).

Patients' clinical symptomatology has to be clearly looked into, considering the mechanical and neurological components. Whole spine standing radiographs, dynamic radiographs, CT, and MRI of the spine have to be taken for proper evaluation. Neural compromise—whether central, lateral, or foraminal—and the cause of stenosis secondary to ligamentum flavum hypertrophy, facets, and/or disc prolapse has to be looked into carefully for deciding the proper procedure. Intervertebral disc height, translation, olisthesis, scoliosis, kyphosis, sagittal balance, lumbosacral angles, pelvic parameters, Cobbs angle of deformities, etc., have to be measured in adult spinal deformities. For example, a patient with lytic grade III spondylolisthesis and radiculopathy with translatory instability and reduced disc height will benefit from OLIF and posterior percutaneous stabilization (**Fig. 2.8**). A patient of degenerative grade I spondylolisthesis and neurogenical claudication with ligamentum flavum hypertrophy will benefit from PLIF. The investigations should also throw light regarding the feasibility of the surgical approach; for example, available space between psoas muscle and the vessels should be more than 8 to 10 mm in OLIF surgeries, level of bifurcation of aorta in ALIF surgeries, anomalous roots like conjoined nerves in PLIF, level of iliac crests and rib cage (**Fig. 2.9**) in DLIF, etc.

Contraindications

The contraindications of lumbar interbody fusion, in general, include severe osteoporosis, where the safety of implants is endangered. The other contraindications are specific to the type of technique used that may complicate/not be feasible for a particular condition. For example, in case of reduced oblique window of <10 mm, OLIF is contraindicated (**Fig. 2.10**).[27] The high-grade spondylolisthesis and reduced disc space are contraindications for MIS-TLIF. Access to the interbody space is problematic and may

Table 2.2 Recommendations based on levels

Options/Levels[a]	T12–L1	L1–2	L2–3	L3–4	L4–5	L5–S1
PLIF	–	++	+++	++++	++++	++++
TLIF	++	++++	++++	++++	++++	++++
DLIF	+++	++++	++++	++++	++++	–
OLIF	–	++	+++	++++	++++	++
ALIF	–	–	++	+++	++++	++++

Abbreviations: ALIF, anterior lumbar interbody fusion; DLIF, direct lumbar interbody fusion; OLIF, oblique lumbar interbody fusion; PLIF, posterior lumbar interbody fusion; TLIF, transforaminal lumbar interbody fusion.
[a]Options—based on feasibility of the approach under assumption of normal sagittal balance.
Note: Limiting factors—PLIF: central cauda equina; DLIF/OLIF: rib cage and Iliac crest; TLIF: nerve roots; ALIF: major vessels.

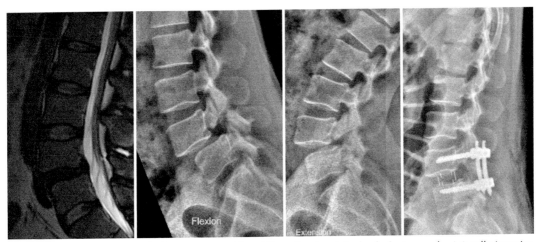

Fig. 2.8 L4–5 lytic spondylolisthesis operated by oblique lumbar interbody fusion and minimally invasive surgery percutaneous pedicle screw fixation.

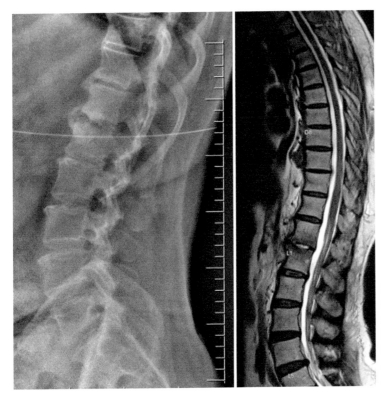

Fig. 2.9 Radiograph of D12–L1 spondylodiscitis with limited access to oblique lumbar interbody fusion/lateral lumbar interbody fusion approach for debridement secondary to rib cage.

end up with significant neurological deficits in PLIF surgeries associated with conjoined root pathologies.[28] Anterior access to the disc space might end up with catastrophic vascular injuries in case of aortic atherosclerosis/aortic aneurysm, retroperitoneal scarring secondary to previous surgery, radiation, etc., and hence ALIF is best avoided in such scenarios.[29]

Conclusion

The most common indications for lumbar interbody fusion are degeneration, infections, developmental pathologies in addition to some extended indications like tumors, trauma, etc. The choice of particular LIF is decided by the

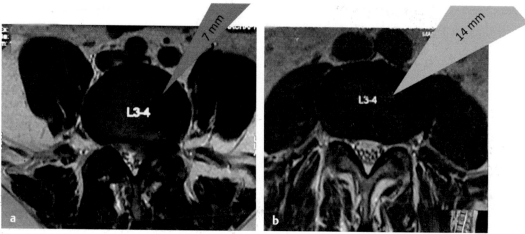

Fig. 2.10 Oblique window—corridor between major vessels and psoas muscle. **(a)** Inadequate (<10 mm)—contraindication for oblique lumbar interbody fusion; **(b)** adequate (>10 mm)—oblique lumbar interbody fusion is possible.

type and level of pathology, including the feasibility of that particular approach. In general, those conditions that require better mechanical correction of bony spine like scoliosis, flat back, or degenerated disc disease-related back pain are better managed by anterior procedures (ALIF/DLIF/OLIF) and those conditions where neural decompression is needed are better dealt with posterior procedures (PLIF/TLIF). Although a preference exists in selecting a particular approach for a specific condition, there has been no clear cut study to prove the superiority of one over another.

Key Points

- TLIF (open/MIS) is the most widely used interbody fusion for various pathologies with satisfactory results.

- ALIF is a viable option for discogenic back-pain and L5–S1 spine pathologies.

- OLIF and LLIF are the best minimally invasive procedures in adult spinal deformity in view of good restoration of spinal balance.

- Circumferential approach is better for revision fusions.

References

1. Derman PB, Albert TJ. Interbody fusion techniques in the surgical management of degenerative lumbar spondylolisthesis. Curr Rev Musculoskelet Med 2017;10(4):530–538

2. Mobbs RJ, Phan K, Malham G, Seex K, Rao PJ. Lumbar interbody fusion: techniques, indications and comparison of interbody fusion options including PLIF, TLIF, MI-TLIF, OLIF/ATP, LLIF and ALIF. J Spine Surg 2015;1(1):2–18

3. Lan T, Hu SY, Zhang YT, et al. Comparison between posterior lumbar interbody fusion and transforaminal lumbar interbody fusion for the treatment of lumbar degenerative diseases: a systematic review and meta-analysis. World Neurosurg 2018;112:86–93

4. Fleege C, Rickert M, Rauschmann M. The PLIF and TLIF techniques. Indication, technique, advantages, and disadvantages [Article in German]. Orthopade 2015;44(2):114–123

5. Sudhir G, Vignesh Jayabalan S, Gadde S, Venkatesh Kumar G, Karthik Kailash K. Analysis of factors influencing ligamentum flavum thickness in lumbar spine: a radiological study of 1070 disc levels in 214 patients. Clin Neurol Neurosurg 2019;182:19–24

6. Sembrano JN, Yson SC, Horazdovsky RD, Santos ER, Polly DW Jr. Radiographic comparison of lateral lumbar interbody fusion versus traditional fusion approaches: analysis of sagittal contour change. Int J Spine Surg 2015;9:16

7. Liu J, Deng H, Long X, et al. A comparative study of perioperative complications between transforaminal versus posterior lumbar interbody fusion in degenerative lumbar spondylolisthesis. Eur Spine J 2016;25(5):1575–1580

8. Zhang Q, Yuan Z, Zhou M, Liu H, Xu Y, Ren Y. A comparison of posterior lumbar interbody fusion and transforaminal lumbar interbody fusion: a literature review and meta-analysis. BMC Musculoskelet Disord 2014;15:367

9. Watkins RG IV, Hanna R, Chang D, Watkins RG III. Sagittal alignment after lumbar interbody fusion: comparing anterior, lateral, and transforaminal approaches. J Spinal Disord Tech 2014;27(5): 253–256

10. Ko MJ, Park SW, Kim YB. Correction of spondylolisthesis by lateral lumbar interbody fusion compared with transforaminal lumbar interbody fusion at L4-5. J Korean Neurosurg Soc 2019; 62(4):422–431

11. Wang J, Zhou Y, Zhang ZF, Li CQ, Zheng WJ, Liu J. Comparison of one-level minimally invasive and open transforaminal lumbar interbody fusion in degenerative and isthmic spondylolisthesis grades 1 and 2. Eur Spine J 2010;19(10):1780–1784

12. Lucio JC, Vanconia RB, Deluzio KJ, Lehmen JA, Rodgers JA, Rodgers W. Economics of less invasive spinal surgery: an analysis of hospital cost differences between open and minimally invasive instrumented spinal fusion procedures during the perioperative period. Risk Manag Healthc Policy 2012;5:65–74

13. Parker SL, Adogwa O, Bydon A, Cheng J, McGirt MJ. Cost-effectiveness of minimally invasive versus open transforaminal lumbar interbody fusion for degenerative spondylolisthesis associated low-back and leg pain over two years. World Neurosurg 2012;78(1-2):178–184

14. Glassman SD, Bridwell K, Dimar JR, Horton W, Berven S, Schwab F. The impact of positive sagittal balance in adult spinal deformity. Spine 2005;30(18):2024–2029

15. Dangelmajer S, Zadnik PL, Rodriguez ST, Gokaslan ZL, Sciubba DM. Minimally invasive spine surgery for adult degenerative lumbar scoliosis. Neurosurg Focus 2014;36(5):E7

16. Manwaring JC, Bach K, Ahmadian AA, Deukmedjian AR, Smith DA, Uribe JS. Management of sagittal balance in adult spinal deformity with minimally invasive anterolateral lumbar interbody fusion: a preliminary radiographic study. J Neurosurg Spine 2014;20(5):515–522

17. Crandall DG, Revella J. Transforaminal lumbar interbody fusion versus anterior lumbar interbody fusion as an adjunct to posterior instrumented correction of degenerative lumbar scoliosis: three year clinical and radiographic outcomes. Spine 2009;34(20):2126–2133

18. Pateder DB, Kebaish KM, Cascio BM, Neubaeur P, Matusz DM, Kostuik JP. Posterior only versus combined anterior and posterior approaches to lumbar scoliosis in adults: a radiographic analysis. Spine 2007;32(14):1551–1554

19. Isaacs RE, Hyde J, Goodrich JA, Rodgers WB, Phillips FM. A prospective, nonrandomized, multicenter evaluation of extreme lateral interbody fusion for the treatment of adult degenerative scoliosis: perioperative outcomes and complications. Spine 2010;35(26, Suppl):S322–S330

20. Choy W, Miller CA, Chan AK, Fu K-M, Park P, Mummaneni PV. Evolution of the minimally invasive spinal deformity surgery algorithm: an evidence-based approach to surgical strategies for deformity correction. Neurosurg Clin North Am 2018;29(3):399–406

21. Sudarshan PK, Suthar HR, Varma VK, Krishnan A, Hegde SK. Long-term experience with reduction technique in high-grade spondylolisthesis in the young. Int J Spine Surg 2018;12(3):399–407

22. Rajakumar DV, Hari A, Krishna M, Sharma A, Reddy M. Complete anatomic reduction and monosegmental fusion for lumbar spondylolisthesis of Grade II and higher: use of the minimally invasive "rocking" technique. Neurosurg Focus 2017;43(2):E12

23. Mobbs RJ, Loganathan A, Yeung V, Rao PJ. Indications for anterior lumbar interbody fusion. Orthop Surg 2013;5(3):153–163

24. Etminan M, Girardi FP, Khan SN, Cammisa FP Jr. Revision strategies for lumbar pseudarthrosis. Orthop Clin North Am 2002;33(2):381–392

25. Lin Y, Li F, Chen W, Zeng H, Chen A, Xiong W. Single-level lumbar pyogenic spondylodiscitis treated with mini-open anterior debridement and fusion in combination with posterior percutaneous fixation via a modified anterior lumbar interbody fusion approach. J Neurosurg Spine 2015;23(6):747–753

26. Shetty AP, Aiyer SN, Kanna RM, Maheswaran A, Rajasekaran S. Pyogenic lumbar spondylodiscitis treated with transforaminal lumbar interbody fusion: safety and outcomes. Int Orthop 2016; 40(6):1163–1170

27. Quillo-Olvera J, Lin GX, Jo HJ, Kim JS. Complications on minimally invasive oblique lumbar interbody fusion at L2-L5 levels: a review of the literature and surgical strategies. Ann Transl Med 2018;6(6):101037

28. Burke SM, Safain MG, Kryzanski J, Riesenburger RI. Nerve root anomalies: implications for transforaminal lumbar interbody fusion surgery and a review of the Neidre and Macnab classification system. Neurosurg Focus 2013;35(2):E9

29. Tannoury T, Kempegowda H, Haddadi K, Tannoury C. Complications associated with minimally invasive anterior to the psoas (ATP) fusion of the lumbosacral spine. Spine 2019. doi: 10.1097/ BRS.0000000000003071. [Epub ahead of print]

Chapter 3

Open Transforaminal Lumbar Interbody Fusion: Overview and Technical Considerations

3 Open Transforaminal Lumbar Interbody Fusion: Overview and Technical Considerations

K. W. Janich, S. N. Kurpad

Introduction

Posterior lumbar interbody fusion (PLIF) was first described by Cloward in 1953,[1] and since then it has had multiple variants described, such as transforaminal, direct lateral, oblique lateral, extreme lateral, anterior, and other variants that further refine a minimally invasive philosophy. Transforaminal lumbar interbody fusion (TLIF) was first described by Harms and Jeszensky in 1998 as a new technique that was made possible by new titanium cage hardware.[2] It was initially motivated by having less retraction on nerve roots. Prospective and retrospective data comparing TLIF with PLIF or posterolateral fusion demonstrates its efficacy with potential for decreased operative times and operative blood loss.[3-5] With recent concerns regarding quality of care, TLIF has also been compared with other forms of fusion regarding cost-effectiveness and found to have similar to better results in this area.[6-8]

Indications

The general indication for TLIF is the requirement for both anterior decompression and fusion. Given this basic form of indication, multiple pathologies have presented themselves in the data as particularly responsive to the procedure.

Patients presenting with radicular symptoms and spinal stenosis in the setting of spondylolisthesis have been shown to do well with operative management, and they do better with fusion rather than decompression alone, especially if back pain is a component of preoperative symptoms.[9] With regard to the approach to fusion, Levin et al showed that TLIF offers better outcomes than posterolateral fusion, though operative time was increased.[10]

Lumbar intervertebral disc pathologies are especially amenable to TLIF. Lateral or foraminal disc herniations require facetectomy or destabilization of the spine otherwise, and in these patients TLIF is a well-studied option. It is also attractive in patients with recurrent disc herniations after initial decompressive surgical management.[11,12] Similarly, disc herniation with back pain due to instability is another pathology amenable to TLIF.

Contraindications

The requirements for destabilization and retraction dictate the anatomic contraindications for TLIF. The primary consideration must be the location on the spinal cord and conus medullaris. While nerve root retraction is a common cause of a temporary radiculopathy or neurological deficit,[5] retraction on the spinal cord or conus can induce a much more devastating permanent deficit. Therefore, the surgeon must consider the location of the conus or the presence of abnormalities, such as tethered cord, prior to committing to this procedure.

Multiple medical contraindications exist and are similar to contraindications for other fusion procedures. Smoking has been shown to significantly increase surgical risks, such as wound dehiscence, blood loss, and pseudoarthrosis.[13-15] Chronic steroid use is associated with adverse outcomes, and the patients using them require frank counselling regarding alternatives to fusion and the increased risk of complications, should fusion be pursued.[16] A similar discussion must be conducted with patients presenting with poor bone quality for any other reason.[17] Caution must be exercised in patients with significant preoperative opioid use, as their pain outcomes tend to be less favorable than patients on a nonopiate chronic pain regimen.[18]

Operative Technique

Preoperative Considerations and Planning

Preoperative instructions for TLIF are similar to those for other lumbar fusion procedures. Ensuring the patient is medically optimized for surgery is the primary concern, but the surgeon also must ensure that procedure-specific risks are minimized. First and foremost, patients must stop smoking prior to the procedure, and laboratory tests—such as for nicotine or carbon monoxide levels—can provide secondary confirmation that this has happened. Patients must also stop taking nonsteroidal anti-inflammatory drugs (NSAIDs) due to the increased risk of pseudoarthrosis and delayed bone healing.[19,20] Many patients regularly take aspirin or another antiplatelet or anticoagulant, and the reason they are on these medications would need to be clarified to determine whether it should be stopped, reduced, or continued through the procedure given its bleeding risks.[21,22]

The key to planning for TLIF is the avoidance of surprises by careful review of the imaging. One of the most important, relevant, and prevalent findings to be aware of is a transitional lumbosacral vertebra to avoid wrong site surgery.[23] Minimizing risk of cerebrospinal fluid leak can be achieved by determining a priori the location of bony defects, especially those from previous lumbar procedures,[24] and their relation to the thecal sac. Knowing the direction and angulation of pedicles in the setting of scoliosis and spondylolisthesis is essential to proper pedicle screw placement. If difficult screw placement is anticipated, consideration should be made to using spinal navigation or fluoroscopy. Neuromonitoring can be considered and is specific for injury,[25] but whether it reduces adverse outcomes is not established at this point.

Anesthesia

General endotracheal anesthesia is the preferred route. Lumbar surgery—generally minimally invasive lumbar surgery—has been performed under monitored anesthesia care or local anesthetic,[26,27] but it would not be recommended for an open TLIF. Sedation and pain control are standard; however, paralytic use will depend on whether the surgeon elects to monitor evoked potentials. A Foley catheter should be placed after induction to monitor volume status and for bladder decompression. Placement of an arterial line will depend on multiple factors, such as local protocols, the anesthesiologist, and surgeon preference. The patient should remain euvolemic and normotensive through the procedure. Due to the location of surgery needing to be below the conus, there is no significant risk to the spinal cord with TLIF; therefore, there is no need to have elevated mean arterial pressures.

Antibiotic Prophylaxis

While no single agent has been shown to be superior over others,[28] the standard regimen in the literature that is reported for preoperative antibiotics is a dose of cefazolin within 1 hour of incision with appropriate redosing as needed—recommended to be every 3 to 4 hours. The antibiotic is generally changed to clindamycin or vancomycin for those with allergies to the penicillins, but this practice has been questioned with evidence of a lack of cross-reactivity[29] and mixed data regarding increased infection rate with alternative regimens.[28] Extended spectrum coverage with vancomycin with or without gram negative coverage is appropriate in complex cases. Similarly, in people with increased wound infection risks, there is evidence supporting intrawound application of vancomycin or gentamicin to decrease the risk.[28,30]

Positioning

The patient is positioned prone in a neutral position with pressure points appropriately padded. The eyes must be checked to ensure there is no pressure placed on them. Goggles, specially designed foam pillows, or skull clamps can assist with positioning the head without pressure on the eyes. In female patients, the breasts must be checked to ensure there is no pressure on them, especially the nipples. The abdomen and genitalia must be allowed to hang free without compression. The patient should be viewed from multiple angles to ensure there is no rotation or other malpositioning.

The lumbar spine should be maintained in its natural lordosis. The complications of fixing the spine in a position out of alignment with this lordosis has been extensively reported in deformity literature, especially as it affects disability and sagittal imbalance.[31,32]

Procedure

After positioning, the incision must be marked. The incision should reflect the length needed to expose the transverse processes of the level above and the level below as well as any area needed for decompression if above or below these levels. Fluoroscopy should be used to localize the incision to avoid exposure of wrong levels. Some choose to mark the incision with ink, while others may choose to scratch the incision to preserve its location after the surgical prep. The area is prepared in a sterile fashion with a chlorhexidine-based scrub[33] and draped with sterile drapes.

Incision is made sharply through the skin and dissection is carried down to the thoracolumbar fascia sharply. Careful hemostasis is maintained at this time to avoid difficulty visualizing anatomy later in the procedure. An optional step is to clear off a shelf of the thoracolumbar fascia to facilitate closure.

The fascia is opened sharply or with electrocautery on top of the spinous processes to be exposed. The subperiosteal plane is maintained as dissection is carried down the spinous process to the lamina, pars, and medial facet. Once the medial facet is encountered, careful separation of planes is warranted to avoid interruption of the joint capsule. The dissection is carried further laterally to the transverse process. Care must be taken to remain in the correct plane to avoid bleeding from nearby pars arteries. If such bleeding is encountered, bipolar electrocautery is quite effective. Often a small portion of the lamina above the expected fusion level needs to be exposed to allow enough lateral retraction to visualize the anatomic landmarks needed to localize the pedicle (**Fig. 3.1**). Levels must be confirmed during the exposure with fluoroscopy.

Fixation is performed in the standard manner. Some surgeons may prefer to perform this process after decompression so instrumentation does not impede bony resection. The cortex is breached with rongeur or drill, and the pedicle is cannulated with a headless awl, Lenke probe, curette, or other preferred instrument (**Fig. 3.2**). The channel must be probed for a breach and, if one is found, the trajectory is adjusted. If the pedicle is sclerotic, the trajectory can be tapped. The pedicle screw is then inserted into the channel, taking care that adequate purchase of the threads is made (**Fig. 3.3**). Depending on surgeon preference, free-handed, fluoroscopically guided, or navigated pedicle screws may be used. Rods must

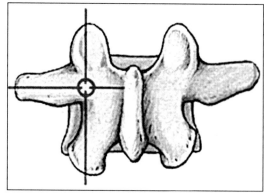

Fig. 3.1 The entry point for pedicle cannulation: the intersection of the middle of the transverse process and pars interarticularis. Reprinted by permission from *Springer Nature: Springer Operative Orthopädie und Traumatologie* "Die posteriore, lumbale, interkorporelle Fusion in unilateraler transforaminaler Technik," Jürgen G. Harms and Dezsö Jeszenszky, 1998.

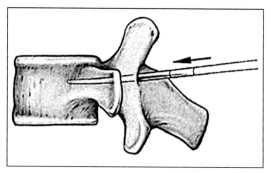

Fig. 3.2 Pedicle cannulation. Reprinted by permission from *Springer Nature: Springer Operative Orthopädie und Traumatologie* "Die posteriore, lumbale, interkorporelle Fusion in unilateraler transforaminaler Technik," Jürgen G. Harms and Dezsö Jeszenszky, 1998.

be sized and bent appropriately to preserve the natural curve of the spine. If reduction of a spondylolisthesis is desired, this step may be performed with reduction screws prior to placement of the interbody graft.

The posterior decompression begins with dissection of the ligamentum flavum from the lamina of the superior level. Removal of the spinous process and lamina is achieved with rongeurs or high-speed drill. Authors have found it advantageous to use a rough diamond bit to achieve hemostasis while drilling. Ensuring that the plane is maintained between the ligamentum flavum and the bone is essential to using drill and rongeurs without causing a cerebrospinal fluid leak. Once the attachment of the ligament is encountered, the dura must be carefully held away from the lamina to complete laminectomy safely. Bony resection is carried laterally to the medial border of the pedicle and superiorly to the top of the lamina.

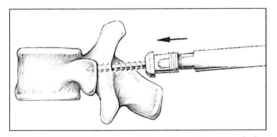

Fig. 3.3 Pedicle screw insertion. Reprinted by permission from *Springer Nature: Springer Operative Orthopädie und Traumatologie* "Die posteriore, lumbale, interkorporelle Fusion in unilateraler transforaminaler Technik," Jürgen G. Harms and Dezsö Jeszenszky, 1998.

Bone must be saved to provide autograft for fusion later in the procedure. The superior portion of the lamina below is also resected in the same fashion to the point needed to provide adequate decompression. The ligament is resected separately or with the bone of the lamina below and laterally.

The pars interarticularis and inferior facet of the superior level are then removed (**Fig. 3.4**). If this bony removal is performed after the laminectomy, the entire ipsilateral nerve root is exposed from axilla to exit from the foramen, allowing it to be protected. The lateral recess can be further decompressed at this point by performing medial facetectomy of the inferior level. The disc space is readily exposed with gentle dissection of the posterior longitudinal ligament with care taken to maintain hemostasis with the nearby epidural venous plexus (**Fig. 3.5**).

The offending disc is localized visually and by palpation. The annulus is incised widely while the root and thecal sac are retracted. The nucleus pulposus is removed (**Fig. 3.6**), and the ipsilateral endplates are cleared of fibrous annulus with a rasp and curettes (**Fig. 3.7**). Care must be taken to expose some cancellous bone not only to facilitate bony fusion but to minimize cortical violation; otherwise graft subsidence will become a significant concern. The end result should be a level surface cleared of soft tissue (**Fig. 3.8**). The interbody graft is sized appropriately such that natural lordosis is preserved and foramina are opened, as undersizing the graft and exaggerated lordosis are associated with radiculopathy and contralateral

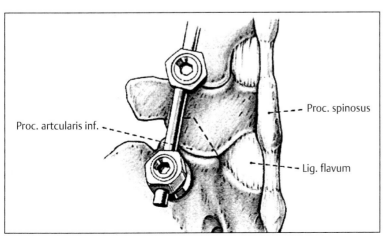

Proc. artcularis inf.

Proc. spinosus

Lig. flavum

Fig. 3.4 The view of the pars interarticularis and inferior articulating process to be removed. Reprinted by permission from *Springer Nature: Springer Operative Orthopädie und Traumatologie* "Die posteriore, lumbale, interkorporelle Fusion in unilateraler transforaminaler Technik," Jürgen G. Harms and Dezsö Jeszenszky, 1998.

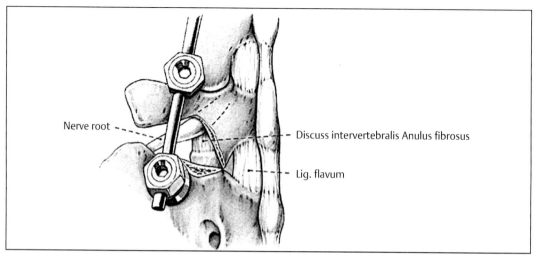

Fig. 3.5 The view of the superior level nerve root and intervertebral disc after resection of the pars inter-articularis, inferior articulating process, and the superior articulating process of the level below. Note that if laminectomy is performed, the nerve root may be visualized to the axilla. Reprinted by permission from *Springer Nature: Springer Operative Orthopädie und Traumatologie* "Die posteriore, lumbale, interkorporelle Fusion in unilateraler transforaminaler Technik," Jürgen G. Harms and Dezsö Jeszenszky, 1998.

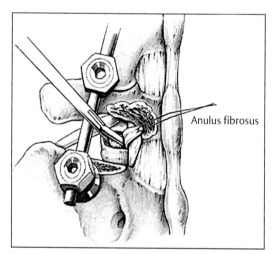

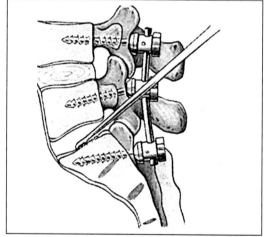

Fig. 3.6 Opening of the annulus fibrosus and resection of nucleus pulposus via pituitary rongeur. Reprinted by permission from *Springer Nature: Springer Operative Orthopädie und Traumatologie* "Die posteriore, lumbale, interkorporelle Fusion in unilateraler transforaminaler Technik," Jürgen G. Harms and Dezsö Jeszenszky, 1998.

Fig. 3.7 Clearing and leveling of the disc space with curettage. Reprinted by permission from *Springer Nature: Springer Operative Orthopädie und Traumatologie* "Die posteriore, lumbale, interkorporelle Fusion in unilateraler transforaminaler Technik," Jürgen G. Harms and Dezsö Jeszenszky, 1998.

foraminal stenosis.[34–36] Autologous bone and fusion adjuncts such as demineralized bone matrix are placed in a cage, and it is positioned in the disc space carefully. If desired, autologous bone can be placed in the remaining disc space to further facilitate fusion (**Fig. 3.9**). Fluoroscopy must be used to confirm the depth of the implant to ensure it is seated deep in the disc space, but not so far forward as to threaten the anterior longitudinal ligament or great vessels.

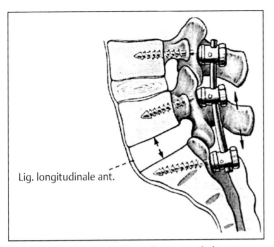

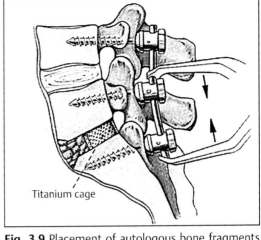

Fig. 3.8 Final appearance of prepared disc space. Reprinted by permission from *Springer Nature: Springer Operative Orthopädie und Traumatologie* "Die posteriore, lumbale, interkorporelle Fusion in unilateraler transforaminaler Technik," Jürgen G. Harms and Dezsö Jeszenszky, 1998.

Fig. 3.9 Placement of autologous bone fragments and cage. Reprinted by permission from *Springer Nature: Springer Operative Orthopädie und Traumatologie* "Die posteriore, lumbale, interkorporelle Fusion in unilateraler transforaminaler Technik," Jürgen G. Harms and Dezsö Jeszenszky, 1998.

A small degree of compression across the interbody graft may be used to facilitate fusion, but caution must be exercised, again, due to a potential for causing foraminal stenosis contralaterally. The rods are then tightened in place to the manufacturer's specification, and the wound is copiously irrigated. The transverse processes and facets of the levels to be fused are decorticated, and autologous bone with or without other fusion adjuncts are placed laterally to facilitate intertransverse fusion (**Fig. 3.10**). Care must be taken to ensure bone chips or other material does not migrate medially or—worse— into the foramen that was just decompressed.

Closure is meticulous and multilayered. While there is some controversy about their usefulness,[37,38,39] there is no prospective data regarding subfascial drains, and consequences to postoperative epidural hematoma can be catastrophic; therefore, authors place a subfascial drain of appropriate size in their TLIF patients. Musculature closure can be performed in layers or in a single layer, ensuring sutures are not so tight so as to cause muscle necrosis. Fascial closure is tight to prevent muscular herniation. Intramuscular bupivacaine can be considered at this point, placed far enough laterally to decrease risk of flow of the anesthetic to the

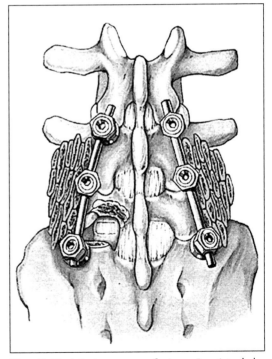

Fig. 3.10 Intertransverse fusion. Reprinted by permission from *Springer Nature: Springer Operative Orthopädie und Traumatologie* "Die posteriore, lumbale, interkorporelle Fusion in unilateraler transforaminaler Technik," Jürgen G. Harms and Dezsö Jeszenszky, 1998.

epidural space.[40] Epifascial antibiotic powder is also placed if desired.[28] If a patient has a satisfactory adipose layer, another layer of suture can bring this portion together or a separate drain can be placed to decrease the size of a postoperative seroma. Dermal sutures are used for a second strength layer. The final layer of skin closure can be performed with a variety of methods. The wound is then covered with a sterile dressing.

The patients are then placed supine in their bed, and anesthesia is reversed. Sometimes symptoms, such as radicular pain, can be assessed immediately upon emergence but others, such as numbness or weakness, will take more time to resolve. The lower extremities must be checked to ensure no new weakness is apparent. If some is present, the distribution must be considered to determine whether it is due to nerve root retraction and potentially temporary or due to another more concerning process requiring further workup.[5]

Postoperative Care

Immediately, postoperative patients should be mobilized once they are able to move. Once the patient mobilizes, consideration consideration may be given for removal of Foley catheter. Physical and occupational therapy are ancillary services that can facilitate safe mobilization and establish criteria for safe discharge to home or the need for further rehabilitation in an inpatient or outpatient facility. Bracing is generally not needed for a single-level fusion but can be considered if a patient falls into one of the high-risk categories for pseudoarthrosis noted previously.

Pain management is always a factor in these cases. Acetaminophen and oral opiates are the mainstay. Muscle relaxants are also provided, with little evidence to support efficacy of one agent over another.[41] Rather, selection of skeletal muscle relaxant may be dictated by potential adverse effects with polypharmacy or the patient's other comorbidities.[42] Consideration can be given to short-term use of NSAIDs, such as ketorolac, but they must be limited or they may risk an increase in nonfusion rates.[43,44] Ketamine has also been a recently used adjunct

for pain control that has been shown to be effective in lumbar surgery, including specifically in patients on chronic opioids.[45,46]

Discharge to home can be achieved once the patient is mobilizing sufficiently to be safe at home, has pain well controlled on oral medications, is tolerating sufficient nutrition and hydration by mouth, and is voiding at his/her baseline. The initial follow-up visit occurs on postoperative day 7 to 10 to reassess the wound and consider suture removal if nonabsorbable suture or staples were used for skin closure. There is variability regarding follow-up frequency and duration, but the authors follow up at 6 weeks and 3 months. If all is well after 3 months, the patient is discharged with plans for follow-up on an as-needed basis.

Conclusion

Open TLIF is a safe, effective, and efficient procedure. The potential advantages of MIS-TLIF (postoperative pain, blood loss) can be replicated quite easily in the open procedure, provided close attention is paid to the dissection technique and surgical anatomy by properly planning each procedure with respect to the choice of indication, patient counseling especially in the preoperative setting, use of imaging to avoid complications, and meticulous surgical technique. Authors routinely discharge patients that undergo open TLIF on the first postoperative day.

Tips and Tricks

- A proper osteotomy cut of lateral facet is the key essential step for insertion of an able-sized cage to prevent future subsidence and pseudoarthrosis.

- Though the approach is unilateral, an adequate disc removal and end plate preparation on the contralateral side is also essential for better fusion rates.

References

1. Cloward RB. The treatment of ruptured lumbar intervertebral discs by vertebral body fusion.

I. Indications, operative technique, after care. J Neurosurg 1953;10(2):154–168

2. Harms JG, Jeszenszky D. Die posteriore, lumbale, interkorporelle Fusion in unilateraler transforaminaler Technik. Oper Orthop Traumatol 1998;10(2):90–102

3. de Kunder SL, van Kuijk SMJ, Rijkers K, et al. Transforaminal lumbar interbody fusion (TLIF) versus posterior lumbar interbody fusion (PLIF) in lumbar spondylolisthesis: a systematic review and meta-analysis. Spine J 2017;17(11):1712–1721

4. Yang EZ, Xu JG, Liu XK, et al. An RCT study comparing the clinical and radiological outcomes with the use of PLIF or TLIF after instrumented reduction in adult isthmic spondylolisthesis. Eur Spine J 2016;25(5):1587–1594

5. Zhang Q, Yuan Z, Zhou M, Liu H, Xu Y, Ren Y. A comparison of posterior lumbar interbody fusion and transforaminal lumbar interbody fusion: a literature review and meta-analysis. BMC Musculoskelet Disord 2014;15:367

6. Bydon M, Macki M, Abt NB, et al. The cost-effectiveness of interbody fusions versus posterolateral fusions in 137 patients with lumbar spondylolisthesis. Spine J 2015;15(3):492–498

7. Kim E, Chotai S, Stonko D, Wick J, Sielatycki A, Devin CJ. A retrospective review comparing two-year patient-reported outcomes, costs, and healthcare resource utilization for TLIF vs. PLF for single-level degenerative spondylolisthesis. Eur Spine J 2018;27(3):661–669

8. Høy K, Bünger C, Niederman B, et al. Transforaminal lumbar interbody fusion (TLIF) versus posterolateral instrumented fusion (PLF) in degenerative lumbar disorders: a randomized clinical trial with 2-year follow-up. Eur Spine J 2013;22(9):2022–2029

9. Ghogawala Z, Dziura J, Butler WE, et al. Laminectomy plus fusion versus laminectomy alone for lumbar spondylolisthesis. N Engl J Med 2016;374(15):1424–1434

10. Levin JM, Tanenbaum JE, Steinmetz MP, Mroz TE, Overley SC. Posterolateral fusion (PLF) versus transforaminal lumbar interbody fusion (TLIF) for spondylolisthesis: a systematic review and meta-analysis. Spine J 2018;18(6):1088–1098

11. Li L, Liu Y, Zhang P, Lei T, Li J, Shen Y. Comparison of posterior lumbar interbody fusion with transforaminal lumbar interbody fusion for treatment of recurrent lumbar disc herniation: a retrospective study. J Int Med Res 2016;44(6):1424–1429

12. Li Z, Tang J, Hou S, et al. Four-year follow-up results of transforaminal lumbar interbody fusion as revision surgery for recurrent lumbar disc herniation after conventional discectomy. J Clin Neurosci 2015;22(2):331–337

13. Echt M, De la Garza Ramos R, Nakhla J, et al. The effect of cigarette smoking on wound complications after single-level posterolateral and interbody fusion for spondylolisthesis. World Neurosurg 2018;116:e824–e829

14. Glassman SD, Anagnost SC, Parker A, Burke D, Johnson JR, Dimar JR. The effect of cigarette smoking and smoking cessation on spinal fusion. Spine 2000;25(20):2608–2615

15. McCunniff PT, Young ES, Ahmadinia K, Ahn UM, Ahn NU. Smoking is associated with increased blood loss and transfusion use after lumbar spinal surgery. Clin Orthop Relat Res 2016;474(4):1019–1025

16. Cloney MB, Garcia RM, Smith ZA, Dahdaleh NS. The effect of steroids on complications, readmission, and reoperation after posterior lumbar fusion. World Neurosurg 2018;110:e526–e533

17. DeWald CJ, Stanley T. Instrumentation-related complications of multilevel fusions for adult spinal deformity patients over age 65: surgical considerations and treatment options in patients with poor bone quality. Spine 2006;31(19, Suppl):S144–S151

18. Villavicencio AT, Nelson EL, Kantha V, Burneikiene S. Prediction based on preoperative opioid use of clinical outcomes after transforaminal lumbar interbody fusions. J Neurosurg Spine 2017;26(2):144–149

19. Dimar JR II, Ante WA, Zhang YP, Glassman SD. The effects of nonsteroidal anti-inflammatory drugs on posterior spinal fusions in the rat. Spine 1996;21(16):1870–1876

20. Allen HL, Wase A, Bear WT. Indomethacin and aspirin: effect of nonsteroidal anti-inflammatory agents on the rate of fracture repair in the rat. Acta Orthop Scand 1980;51(4):595–600

21. Kang SB, Cho KJ, Moon KH, Jung JH, Jung SJ. Does low-dose aspirin increase blood loss after spinal fusion surgery? Spine J 2011;11(4):303–307

22. Park HJ, Kwon KY, Woo JH. Comparison of blood loss according to use of aspirin in lumbar fusion patients. Eur Spine J 2014;23(8):1777–1782

23. Lian J, Levine N, Cho W. A review of lumbosacral transitional vertebrae and associated vertebral numeration. Eur Spine J 2018;27(5):995–1004

24. Ghobrial GM, Theofanis T, Darden BV, Arnold P, Fehlings MG, Harrop JS. Unintended durotomy in lumbar degenerative spinal surgery: a 10-year systematic review of the literature. Neurosurg Focus 2015;39(4):E8

25. Melachuri SR, Kaur J, Melachuri MK, et al. The diagnostic accuracy of somatosensory evoked potentials in evaluating neurological deficits during 1057 lumbar interbody fusions. J Clin Neurosci 2019;61:78–83

26. Kim KH. Safe sedation and hypnosis using dexmedetomidine for minimally invasive spine

surgery in a prone position. Korean J Pain 2014; 27(4):313–320

27. Sairyo K, Chikawa T, Nagamachi A. State-of-the-art transforaminal percutaneous endoscopic lumbar surgery under local anesthesia: discectomy, foraminoplasty, and ventral facetectomy. J Orthop Sci 2018;23(2):229–236

28. Shaffer WO, Baisden JL, Fernand R, Matz PG; North American Spine Society. An evidence-based clinical guideline for antibiotic prophylaxis in spine surgery. Spine J 2013;13(10):1387–1392

29. Campagna JD, Bond MC, Schabelman E, Hayes BD. The use of cephalosporins in penicillin-allergic patients: a literature review. J Emerg Med 2012; 42(5):612–620

30. Sweet FA, Roh M, Sliva C. Intrawound application of vancomycin for prophylaxis in instrumented thoracolumbar fusions: efficacy, drug levels, and patient outcomes. Spine 2011;36(24):2084–2088

31. Potter BK, Lenke LG, Kuklo TR. Prevention and management of iatrogenic flatback deformity. J Bone Joint Surg Am 2004;86(8):1793–1808

32. Boody BS, Rosenthal BD, Jenkins TJ, Patel AA, Savage JW, Hsu WK. Iatrogenic llatback and flatback syndrome: evaluation, management, and prevention. Clin Spine Surg 2017;30(4):142–149

33. Darouiche RO, Wall MJ Jr, Itani KM, et al. Chlorhexidine-alcohol versus povidone-iodine for surgical-site antisepsis. N Engl J Med 2010; 362(1):18–26

34. Hunt T, Shen FH, Shaffrey CI, Arlet V. Contralateral radiculopathy after transforaminal lumbar interbody fusion. Eur Spine J 2007;16(Suppl 3): 311–314

35. Iwata T, Miyamoto K, Hioki A, Fushimi K, Ohno T, Shimizu K. Morphologic changes in contralateral lumbar foramen in unilateral cantilever transforaminal lumbar interbody fusion using kidney-type intervertebral spacers. J Spinal Disord Tech 2015;28(5):E270–E276

36. Jang KM, Park SW, Kim YB, Park YS, Nam TK, Lee YS. Acute contralateral radiculopathy after unilateral transforaminal lumbar interbody fusion. J Korean Neurosurg Soc 2015;58(4):350–356

37. Chimenti P, Molinari R. Post-operative spinal epidural hematoma causing American Spinal Injury Association B spinal cord injury in patients with suction wound drains. J Spinal Cord Med 2013;36(3):213–219

38. Choi HS, Lee SG, Kim WK, Son S, Jeong TS. Is surgical drain useful for lumbar disc surgery? Korean J Spine 2016;13(1):20–23

39. Kou J, Fischgrund J, Biddinger A, Herkowitz H. Risk factors for spinal epidural hematoma after spinal surgery. Spine 2002;27(15):1670–1673

40. Perera AP, Chari A, Kostusiak M, Khan AA, Luoma AM, Casey ATH. Intramuscular local anesthetic infiltration at closure for postoperative analgesia in lumbar spine surgery: a systematic review and meta-analysis. Spine 2017;42(14):1088–1095

41. Chou R, Peterson K, Helfand M. Comparative efficacy and safety of skeletal muscle relaxants for spasticity and musculoskeletal conditions: a systematic review. J Pain Symptom Manage 2004;28(2):140–175

42. Lamberg JJ, Gordin VN. Serotonin syndrome in a patient with chronic pain polypharmacy. Pain Med 2014;15(8):1429–1431

43. Pradhan BB, Tatsumi RL, Gallina J, Kuhns CA, Wang JC, Dawson EG. Ketorolac and spinal fusion: does the perioperative use of ketorolac really inhibit spinal fusion? Spine 2008;33(19):2079–2082

44. Glassman SD, Rose SM, Dimar JR, Puno RM, Campbell MJ, Johnson JR. The effect of post-operative nonsteroidal anti-inflammatory drug administration on spinal fusion. Spine 1998; 23(7):834–838

45. Nielsen RV, Fomsgaard JS, Siegel H, et al. Intraoperative ketamine reduces immediate postoperative opioid consumption after spinal fusion surgery in chronic pain patients with opioid dependency: a randomized, blinded trial. Pain 2017;158(3):463–470

46. Brinck EC, Tiippana E, Heesen M, et al. Perioperative intravenous ketamine for acute postoperative pain in adults. Cochrane Database Syst Rev 2018;12:CD012033

Chapter 4

Minimally Invasive Surgical Transforaminal Lumbar Interbody Fusion

4 Minimally Invasive Surgical Transforaminal Lumbar Interbody Fusion

Satish Rudrappa, Ramachandran Govindasamy, T. V. Ramakrishna

Introduction

Harms and Rolinger revolutionized inter-body fusion by approaching via transforaminal route, in 1982, to combat the complication of significant nerve and thecal sac retraction associated with posterior approach.[1] In transforaminal lumbar interbody fusion (TLIF), the disc is approached through lateral access with very minimal retraction. The clinical and radiological outcomes of these open procedures are satisfactory, but at the cost of extensive paraspinal muscle dissection and retraction. In 2002, Foley et al, introduced the concept of minimally invasive surgery (MIS) for performing the TLIF procedure, in an attempt to reduce the limitations associated with conventional open TLIF.[2]

In MIS-TLIF, a paramedian incision is made and the disc space is reached through natural anatomical planes. This technique reduces the muscle dissection and retraction, thereby significantly limiting the chance of iatrogenic damage and muscle atrophy.[3,4,5,6,7] The added advantages in MIS-TLIF include less blood loss, reduced postoperative pain and infection, early hospital recovery, and shorter stay.[8,9] The advent of instruments and navigation techniques in spine surgeries have popularized MIS-TLIF in recent days. In the current scenario, MIS-TLIF depicts use of tubular system to perform the interbody fusion and percutaneous pedicle screw (PPS) instrumentation for optimal results. However, this requires a long learning curve.[10] In this chapter, the authors intend to discuss the indications, preoperative planning, surgical techniques, results, and complications associated with MIS-TLIF.

Indications

The surgical indication of performing an LIF at all levels from L1–L2 to L5–S1 can be addressed by MIS-TLIF, provided there is adequate armamentarium and expertise in the technique. The common indications are low-grade spondylolisthesis, degenerative lumbar canal stenosis with or without scoliosis, disc prolapse, spondylodiscitis, etc. However, high-grade spondylolisthesis (> 50%) and osteoporosis are relative contraindications for MIS, as the technical feasibility in reducing the slip is not yet studied completely.[11]

Preoperative Planning

For a successful surgical technique, preoperative planning including clinical and radiological evaluation is crucial. Patient with unilateral radiculopathy is the most common presentation in lumbar degenerative disease and also the ideal candidate for surgical management by MIS-TLIF procedure. The identification of the contralateral exiting nerve root is challenging and in exceptional cases, with significant bilateral pathology, might require MIS approach.[12] The patients are investigated with anteroposterior and lateral X-rays, magnetic resonance imaging (MRI), and computed tomography (CT) when needed. Standing whole-spine and dynamic radiographs of lumbar spine help in identifying the disc height, coronal and sagittal balance, translatory slips, lumbosacral kyphosis, pedicle sizes, etc. Preoperative planning should also include the assessment of pedicle diameter especially in dysplastic spondylolisthesis (L5–S1). CT is done selectively to look for size of pedicles in dysplastic listhesis and previous laminectomy defects. Special attention should be given to facet hypertrophy, ligamentum flavum thickening, lateral recess stenosis, and anomalous nerve roots such as conjoint/furcal roots in MRI. When the clinical history and presentation correlates well with the radiological findings, patient outcomes will be excellent.

Surgical Anatomy

The muscles present in the posterior lumbar spine are arranged in layers.[13] Latissimus dorsi and thoracolumbar fascia are superficially placed with multifidus and rotator muscles located deep. The lower back muscles are (from ventral to dorsal) quadratus lumborum, erector spinae, and multifidus which helps in maintaining the lordosis of lumbar spine. This lordosis reduces the effects of gravity on spine, and it is a unique phenomenon observed only in human beings. Any change in this lordosis increases the load on lumbar disc leading to degeneration and back pain. The paramedian natural plane is between the multifidus and longissimus part of erector spinae muscle through which the tubes are passed[14] (**Fig. 4.1**). The advantage of MIS approach over open procedures in revision cases is because of this plane as it avoids the previous midline scar and laminectomy defects. This also spares the natural tension band of the posterior spine and also preserves the muscles on the contralateral side with minimal damage on the side of the procedure. The working corridor in TLIF is "Kambin's" triangle bound by thecal sac with traversing nerve root medially

and exiting root with cephalad vertebra superiorly. The inferior border is made by the superior pedicle margin of the caudal vertebra.

Surgical Steps

Operative Setup

Patient is positioned prone on a radiolucent table over the bolsters (to enhance lordosis) in such a way that there is no increase in intra-abdominal pressure. Arms are rested in abduction (90 degrees) and placed on both the sides with legs in mild knee flexion. Pressure points are adequately taken care of and electrode placement for neural monitoring is done appropriately according to the level of the surgeon so as to assess any potential changes that may occur during the surgical procedure. Electromyography (EMG) monitoring is more useful during the pedicle screw placements. Head is positioned on a hood or on head pins, fixed to Sugitha/Mayfield frames (**Fig. 4.2**). Pins have certain advantages, as hoods are associated with increased pressure on the eyes, facial edema, lip injuries, and soft-tissue abrasions.

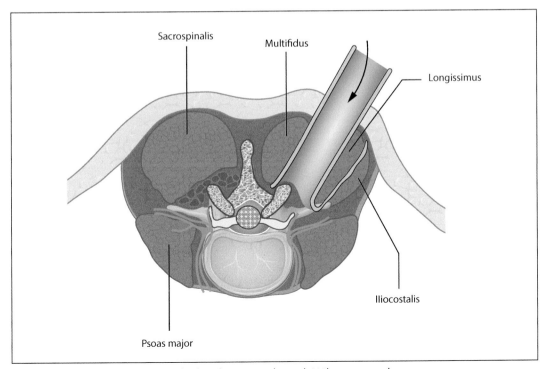

Fig. 4.1 Pictorial representation of tube placement through Wiltse approach.

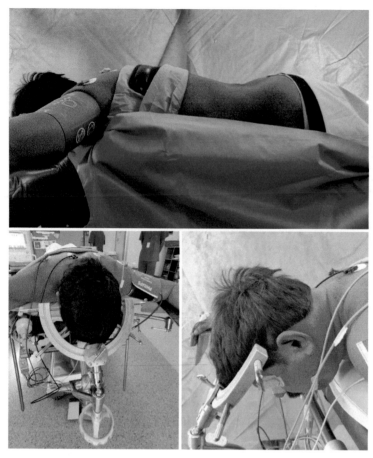

Fig. 4.2 Positioning the patient with head fixed on a Sugitha pin frame.

These should be avoided especially when monitoring motor-evoked potentials (MEPs), which produce significant motion.

Surgical Technique

MIS-TLIF consists of four important sequential steps which are as follows:

1. PPS insertion and rod application.
2. Neural decompression through the tubes.
3. Discectomy and end plate preparation.
4. Cage placement.

Percutaneous Pedicle Screw Placement and Rod Application

The pedicles contralateral to the side of the decompression are instrumented first and then rod is applied. The method of inserting PPS is mainly based on the type of imaging that can be obtained intraoperatively. These include fluoroscopy-/navigation-based intraoperative imaging (C-arm/Iso 3D/CT). In a fluoroscopy-based image setting, a proper anteroposterior radiograph is compulsory with no parallax errors. An ideal anteroposterior radiograph should show parallel end plates with pedicles visualized equally on both sides and spinous process in the midline (**Fig. 4.3**). Once the radiograph is obtained, three parallel lines are made on the skin surface: one along the midline spinous process and two along the lateral border of both pedicles (**Fig. 4.3**). A stab incision of 2 cm (more lateral in case of obese patients) is made just lateral to the lateral border of the pedicle and Jamshidi needle is advanced until the transverse process and facet junction are reached. A starting point is made at 10'o clock (right) or 2'o clock (left) position of the pedicle (**Fig. 4.4a**) and further advanced at increments of 5 mm in desirable angles slowly until the medial wall of the pedicle is reached (**Fig. 4.4b**). All these

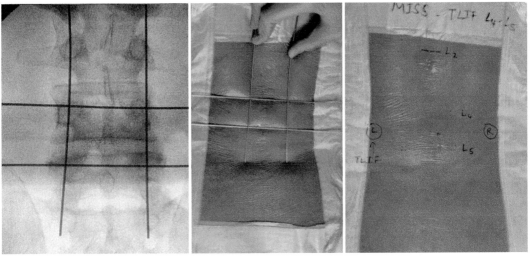

Fig. 4.3 Colinear fluoroscopic image showing linear end plate and skin marking corresponding to the lateral border of pedicles.

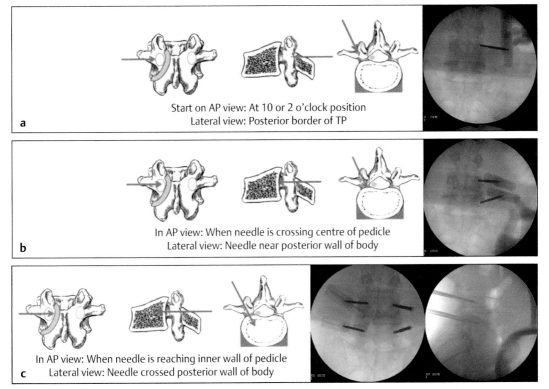

a Start on AP view: At 10 or 2 o'clock position
Lateral view: Posterior border of TP

b In AP view: When needle is crossing centre of pedicle
Lateral view: Needle near posterior wall of body

c In AP view: When needle is reaching inner wall of pedicle
Lateral view: Needle crossed posterior wall of body

Fig. 4.4 Serial images of Jamshidi needle insertion position for pedicle screw preparation **(a)** at entry point, **(b)** at mid-pedicle, and **(c)** crossing the medial pedicle wall into vertebral body.

should be monitored carefully under anteroposterior fluoroscopy. It is followed by lateral fluoroscopy imaging to demonstrate the position of the needle tip, which should be anterior to the pedicle–vertebral body junction (**Fig. 4.4c**).

If the Jamshidi tip position has not reached the vertebral body, further advancement of the needle might lead to medial pedicular breach. The Jamshidi needles are then replaced by guide wires and fenestrated pedicle screws of adequate length and size, which are advanced after serial tapping on the contralateral (opposite of TLIF) side (**Fig. 4.5**). Serial lateral imaging is must to avoid inadvertent migration of the guide wire anteriorly into the abdomen.

Caution should be taken in advancing the pedicle screws as the tulips of cranial and caudal screws should be at same levels, viz anteroposterior/mediolateral, for easy placement of the rods. The rod is then inserted into the pedicle screws and cannulation of the ipsilateral pedicles are performed as described before with the guide wires left in situ (**Fig. 4.6**). The advantage of using navigation is better identification of the pedicles with significantly less radiation exposure consuming less time. It also helps in teaching purpose and is better compared with fluoroscopy-based PPS placements.

Neural Decompression through Tubes

MIS-TLIF involves mastering the technique to work within the narrow portal tubes and in vicinity of neural elements. To achieve an adequate decompression of nerve roots, proper docking of the tubes is the first priority. A guide wire has to be placed at the level of facet undergoing removal, followed by sequential passage of tubes to dilate the muscles. Authors prefer to place 22-mm-diameter tubes of appropriate depth to decompress the neural canal (**Fig. 4.7**). A properly docked tube should make visualization of the important bony elements easy. This includes pars interarticularis cranially, medial facet laterally, spinolaminar junction medially, and the superior border of caudal lamina

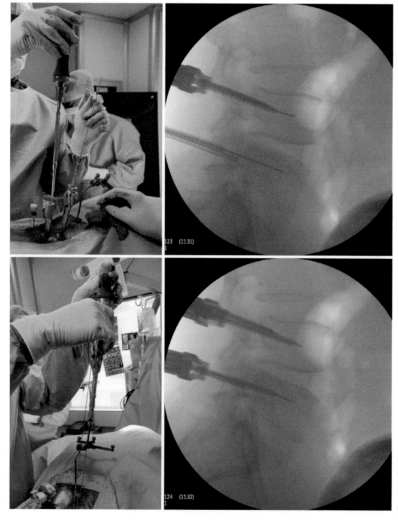

Fig. 4.5 Pedicle preparation with serial tapping followed by screw insertion over guide wires.

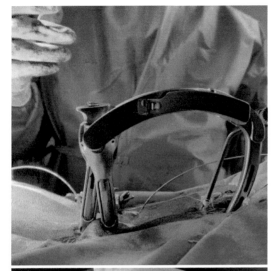

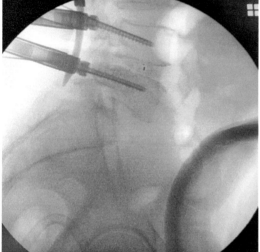

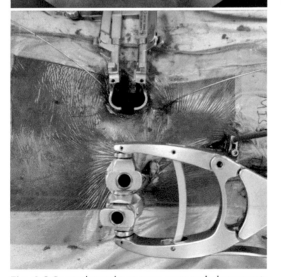

Fig. 4.6 Contralateral percutaneous rod placement; bent guide wires on ipsilateral side after tapping.

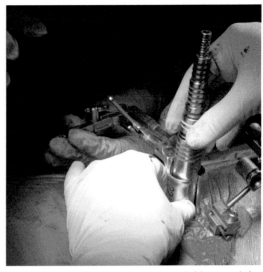

Fig. 4.7 Tube placement after serial dilation of the Wiltse plane.

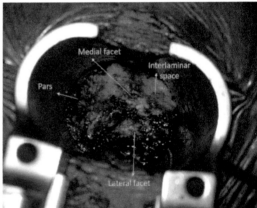

Fig. 4.8 Visualization of bony elements through properly docked tubes.

inferiorly (**Fig. 4.8**). Some residual muscles and soft tissue are removed by monopolar cautery and pituitary forceps.

Authors prefer to osteotomize at the pars interarticularis level and spinolaminar junction to harvest the medial facet that can be used as a bone graft to fill the interbody cage. The alternate methods include use of high-speed burr or Kerrison rongeur. Once the medial facetectomy is complete, superior and medial portion of lateral facet are removed for adequate exposure (**Figs. 4.9 and 4.10**). The bony spikes left off after osteotomies are cleared off using Kerrison rongeur before exposing the neural structures covered by ligamentum flavum.

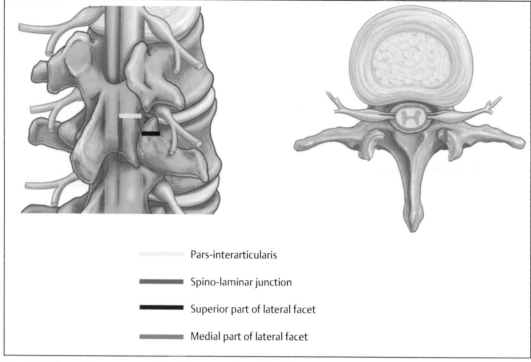

Pars-interarticularis

Spino-laminar junction

Superior part of lateral facet

Medial part of lateral facet

Fig. 4.9 Schematic representation of osteotomies of the facets.

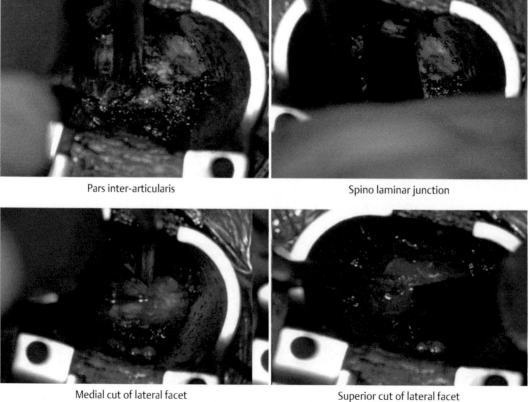

Pars inter-articularis

Spino laminar junction

Medial cut of lateral facet

Superior cut of lateral facet

Fig. 4.10 Microscopic images of serial facet osteotomies.

Authors routinely prefer operating micro- scope to clear off the ligamentum flavum in central and lateral recess. The microscope along with the tubes can be tilted to complete the contralateral flavectomy by "over-the-top decompression" method. Using this method, the nerve roots on the opposite side can be visu- alized and cleared. The operating microscope helps in identifying and coagulating epidural veins, preserving epidural fat, identification of ipsilateral exiting, traversing roots, and con- tralateral traversing root clearly. Surgical loupes with adequate light source might do the same job and are preferred by some surgeons.

Discectomy and End Plate Preparation

The interbody disc space is identified through the Kambin's triangle with adequate control of epidural venous plexus followed by incision of posterolateral annulus to complete the dis- cectomy (**Fig. 4.11**). Judicious use of Kerrison rongeurs at this stage will help in widening the annulotomy defect to reach the contralateral side of the disc without damaging the neural structures. A subtotal discectomy is completed by using the combination of specialized instru- ments such as disc shavers, pituitary rongeurs, and curettes (**Fig. 4.12**). End plates are prepared with paddle distractors, shavers, and curettes. The typical gritty feel of the end plates is the indicator of optimal fusion bed. Adequate end plate preparation is the key for successful TLIF surgery especially in MIS procedures as the available autografts are less. End plate prepara- tion should be carefully done in case of osteopo- rosis as there is a high chance of cage migration into the body secondary to end plate fractures.

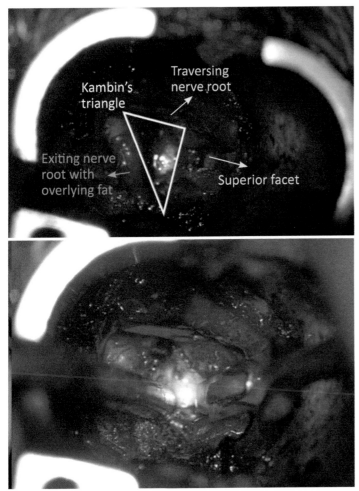

Fig. 4.11 Microscopic demon- stration of Kambin's triangle and annulotomy of disc.

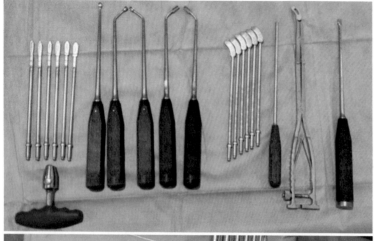

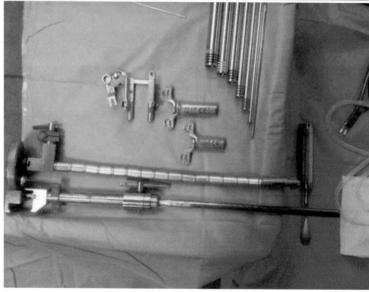

Fig. 4.12 Instrumentation required for interbody workup, including minimally invasive surgery tubes.

Cage Placement

Trial interbody cages of various sizes are provided with the cage system, and appropriate size and height of the cage should be chosen to produce adequate lordosis. A slight distraction of the intervertebral space will be useful at this stage using the pedicle screws placed contralaterally to choose a larger cage (indirect decompression of the exiting roots). After confirmation with lateral fluoroscopic imaging, the disc space is irrigated to remove the loose disc fragments and morselized bone autografts are placed in the anterior third of disc space in a tight fashion. Authors prefer to use bean-shaped or banana-shaped polyether ether ketone (PEEK) cage packed with autografts.

The autografts are derived from the spinolaminar bones that has osteogenic, osteoconductive, and osteoinductive potential for good fusion. The banana-shaped TLIF cage is inserted carefully with gentle retraction of the traversing root and placed at anterior third of disc space farthest from pedicle screw construct in midline (**Fig. 4.13**). This gives stability in lateral bending as well as in flexion-extension planes.[15,16,17] The final position of the cage is confirmed by fluoroscopy and the distraction is released on the contralateral side. The pedicle screws are then applied on to the cannulated pedicles using guide wires and the rods are applied in compression mode followed by final fluoroscopy to confirm position of all implants (**Fig. 4.14**). The wound is irrigated and closure is done in layers.

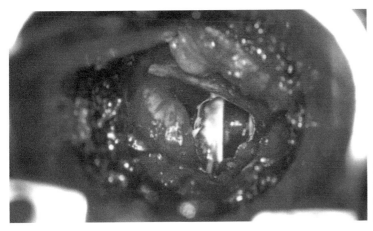

Fig. 4.13 Microscopic picture demonstrating the final position of the transforaminal lumbar interbody fusion cage.

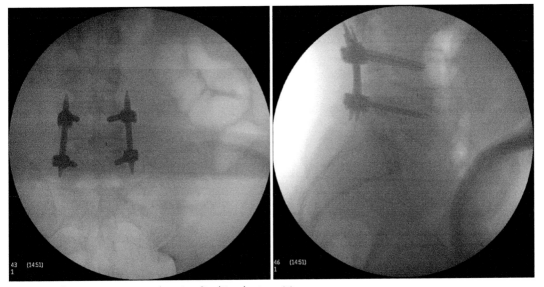

Fig. 4.14 Fluoroscopy image showing final implant position.

Outcomes and Review of Literature

In conventional open procedures the iatrogenic muscle damage, especially multifidus, is more—leading to poor operative outcome measures. These muscle damages are demonstrated by increase in creatine phosphokinase (CPK) levels, and postoperative MRI changes.[18] MIS-TLIF significantly avoids this damage as it goes through the anatomical planes without damaging the muscles. Placement of the pedicle screws through anatomical plane via MIS approach is associated with less blood loss, lesser muscle damage, lesser postoperative pain, lesser use of narcotics, early mobilization, and shortened hospital stay.[19] The average duration of MIS-TLIF surgery ranges from 120 minutes for a single level to 360 minutes for multiple levels, which is comparable to 142–312 minutes in an open procedure.[20–23]

The average blood loss is significantly lower in MIS-TLIF group (226 mL) as against open (1,147 mL) group.[24] The surgical site infections are less compared with open procedures owing to less tissue damage in MIS-TLIF. In recent years, advancements in surgical expertise and instrumentation have led to comparable fusion rates between MIS-TLIF (93.4%) and open procedures (93.8%).[25] The placement of PPS is safe and the misplacement rates are comparable to open TLIF. Smith et al[26] demonstrated 6.2% pedicle breaches in a CT-based study of 601 patients and 2/37 breaches were symptomatic.

Complications

Dural Tears

The incidence of accidental durotomy ranges between 1.8 and 13.9%,[27] and is more common in obese patients and revision surgeries. It can happen specifically during cage placement or neural decompression. Small dural tears rarely need any repair as they are less likely to cause significant or persistent cerebrospinal fluid leak owing to lack of dead space when the muscles fall back on removal of the tubes. However, large dural tears with exteriorization of root(s) may need conversion to open procedure and repositioning the root(s). However, all cases with dural tears can be mobilized comfortably on first postoperative day.

Pedicle Screw and Rod Misplacement

Malposition of the pedicle screw can occur due to improper visualization of entry point, and can cause significant morbidity such as impingement of the exiting nerve following inferior breach and neural compression following medial breach. It can be best avoided by good intraoperative imaging (colinear X-rays, vigilance for medial wall breach). Navigation system has proven to be effective in increasing accuracy of screw placement.[28] Intraoperative identification of malpositioned screws can most often be managed without conversion to open procedure. Postoperative identification of malposition producing radiculopathy needs revision of the screw.[29]

Nerve Root Injuries

The reported incidence of nerve root injuries is 3.2%.[30] It can occur by involving the traversing root during decompression or cage placement and is often transient with good recovery unless the nerve root is completely severed.[30]

Exiting nerve root injuries occur rarely if the roots are low lying.

Radiation Hazard

High radiation exposure following fluoroscopy-assisted MIS-TLIF is well established (2.93 Gy/cm^2), especially in the surgeons who are beginners and it can be considerably reduced by using navigation assistance (0.47 Gy/cm^2).[31]

Cage-Related Problems

Insufficient access to the disc space can result in the cage getting stuck during insertion or may result in making a surgeon use a smaller cage which is prone to migrate or cause pseudoarthrosis. The access can be improved by osteotomizing a part of superior (lateral) facet and applying contralateral distraction by rods. Cage migration is not very uncommon and is reported up to 1.2%.[32] It is more common with smaller, rectangular cage and in patients with flat rather than concave end plates.[32] Posterior migration can cause severe neurological deficit and warrants open revision.

Tips and Tricks

PPS Placement and Rod Application

For a successful PPS placement, proper anteroposterior fluoroscopy demonstrating "bulls eye view" of the targeted pedicle is a must and any concerns should prompt for an open surgery. Authors prefer to cannulate all pedicles using anteroposterior fluoroscopy by two independent surgeons before proceeding to lateral imaging confirming the final position. This reduces the time taken and radiation exposure significantly. A full control of the guide wire is essential to prevent forward advancement (risk of damage to gut, vessels, and intra-abdominal contents) or inadvertent dislodgement of guide wires especially during tapping. At the L5–S1 level, L5 and S1 pedicle screw sleeves can impinge each other at the level of skin which can be avoided by placing the S1 screw little caudally.[33]

Rods of appropriate length and contour have to be selected as the removal of rods after application is not always easy. Multiple skin incisions lined up for multiple segment fixations represent an easier aspect of rod insertion. In cases with scoliosis, rod application might be difficult even in experienced hands. During insertion, palpable engagement is tested by rod tester and confirmed by radiographs—anteroposterior, lateral, and oblique—as single level imaging might be deceptive at times (**Fig. 4.15**). In case of a difficulty arising in passing the rods through the tulips of all screws in a multilevel instrumentation setup, it is advised to do further advancement or withdrawal of the pedicle screws. This is to attain levelling of all the tulips and in addition keeping the screws polyaxial without getting it fixed to the facets. Despite doing all these adjustments, passage of the rods might be still difficult at times and may end up in connecting the adjacent skin incisions making it an open procedure. In case of systems such as Sextant (Medtronic Inc., Memphis), the prebent lordotic rods can be troublesome in patients with kyphosis.

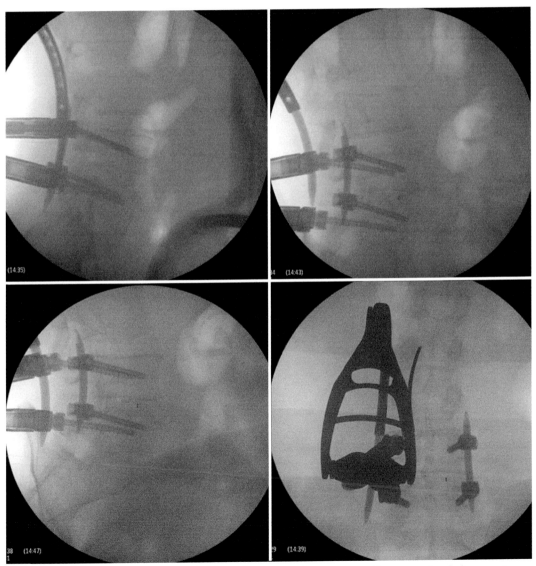

Fig. 4.15 Anteroposterior, lateral, and oblique fluoroscopy images to confirm correct rod placement.

Decompression and Interbody Fusion

The proper positioning of tubes is a must for successful decompression and interbody workup.[34] The tubes are placed over the facet joint with trajectory parallel to the disc space that has to be confirmed by imaging before proceeding. A complete facetectomy extending from pars to spinolaminar junction is a must to get an adequate window. A short vertical window might end up in excess retraction of the thecal sac resulting in dural and nerve injuries. When the exiting nerve root is located more inferiorly, an extra resection of the lateral facet at superior margins will reduce the manipulation of that root. A contralateral "over-the-top" decompression before discectomy will ease in retraction of the dural sac. Adequate removal of the medial side of the lateral facet will aid in placing a larger-sized cage.

Conclusion

The MIS-TLIF is a safe and effective method among all other LIF procedures having lesser iatrogenic muscle damage. However, a steep learning curve is required for the spinal surgeons to master this technique to get optimal results. A thorough understanding of the surgical anatomy through tubes and stepwise approach is essential for a successful procedure. However, conversion to an open TLIF should be considered at times in the event of any associated complications.

References

1. Harms J, Rolinger H. A one-stager procedure in operative treatment of spondylolistheses: dorsal traction-reposition and anterior fusion (author's transl). [in German] Z Orthop Ihre Grenzgeb 1982;120(3):343–347
2. Foley KT, Holly LT, Schwender JD. Minimally invasive lumbar fusion. Spine 2003;28(15, Suppl): S26–S35
3. Datta G, Gnanalingham KK, Peterson D, et al. Back pain and disability after lumbar laminectomy: is there a relationship to muscle retraction? Neurosurgery 2004;54(6):1413–1420, discussion 1420
4. Gejo R, Matsui H, Kawaguchi Y, Ishihara H, Tsuji H. Serial changes in trunk muscle performance after posterior lumbar surgery. Spine 1999;24(10): 1023–1028
5. Kawaguchi Y, Matsui H, Tsuji H. Back muscle injury after posterior lumbar spine surgery. Part 1: Histologic and histochemical analyses in rats. Spine 1994;19(22):2590–2597
6. Sihvonen T, Herno A, Paljärvi L, Airaksinen O, Partanen J, Tapaninaho A. Local denervation atrophy of paraspinal muscles in postoperative failed back syndrome. Spine 1993;18(5):575–581
7. Styf JR, Willén J. The effects of external compression by three different retractors on pressure in the erector spine muscles during and after posterior lumbar spine surgery in humans. Spine 1998;23(3):354–358
8. Kim K-T, Lee S-H, Suk K-S, Bae S-C. The quantitative analysis of tissue injury markers after mini-open lumbar fusion. Spine 2006;31(6):712–716
9. Schwender JD, Holly LT, Rouben DP, Foley KT. Minimally invasive transforaminal lumbar interbody fusion (TLIF): technical feasibility and initial results. J Spinal Disord Tech 2005;18(1, Suppl): S1–S6
10. Peng CW, Yue WM, Poh SY, Yeo W, Tan SB. Clinical and radiological outcomes of minimally invasive versus open transforaminal lumbar interbody fusion. Spine 2009;34(13):1385–1389
11. Rajakumar DV, Hari A, Krishna M, Sharma A, Reddy M. Complete anatomic reduction and monosegmental fusion for lumbar spondylolisthesis of Grade II and higher: use of the minimally invasive "rocking" technique. Neurosurg Focus 2017;43(2):E12
12. Lee CK, Park JY, Zhang HY. Minimally invasive transforaminal lumbar interbody fusion using a single interbody cage and a tubular retraction system: technical tips, and perioperative, radiologic and clinical outcomes. J Korean Neurosurg Soc 2010;48(3):219–224
13. Creze M, Soubeyrand M, Gagey O. The paraspinal muscle-tendon system: Its paradoxical anatomy. PLoS One 2019;14(4):e0214812
14. Guiroy A, Sícoli A, Masanés NG, Ciancio AM, Gagliardi M, Falavigna A. How to perform the Wiltse posterolateral spinal approach: Technical note. Surg Neurol Int 2018;9:38
15. Quigley KJ, Alander DH, Bledsoe JG. An in vitro biomechanical investigation: variable positioning of leopard carbon fiber interbody cages. J Spinal Disord Tech 2008;21(6):442–447
16. Kwon BK, Berta S, Daffner SD, et al. Radiographic analysis of transforaminal lumbar interbody fusion for the treatment of adult isthmic spondylolisthesis. J Spinal Disord Tech 2003;16(5): 469–476

17. Bono CM, Khandha A, Vadapalli S, Holekamp S, Goel VK, Garfin SR. Residual sagittal motion after lumbar fusion: a finite element analysis with implications on radiographic flexion-extension criteria. Spine 2007;32(4):417–422

18. Lombao Iglesias D, Bagó Granell J, Vilor Rivero T. Validity of creatine kinase as an indicator of muscle injury in spine surgery and its relation with postoperative pain. Acta Orthop Belg 2014; 80(4):545–550

19. Patel DV, Bawa MS, Haws BE, et al. PROMIS Physical Function for prediction of postoperative pain, narcotics consumption, and patient-reported outcomes following minimally invasive transforaminal lumbar interbody fusion. J Neurosurg Spine 2019;:1–7; Epub ahead of print. doi: 10.3171/2018.9.SPINE18863

20. Villavicencio AT, Burneikiene S, Roeca CM, Nelson EL, Mason A. Minimally invasive versus open transforaminal lumbar interbody fusion. Surg Neurol Int 2010;1:12–22

21. Shunwu F, Xing Z, Fengdong Z, Xiangqian F. Minimally invasive transforaminal lumbar inter-body fusion for the treatment of degenerative lumbar diseases. Spine 2010;35(17):1615–1620

22. Wang J, Zhou Y, Zhang ZF, Li CQ, Zheng WJ, Liu J. Comparison of one-level minimally invasive and open transforaminal lumbar interbody fusion in degenerative and isthmic spondylolisthesis grades 1 and 2. Eur Spine J 2010;19(10):1780–1784

23. Isaacs RE, Podichetty VK, Santiago P, et al. Minimally invasive microendoscopy-assisted transforaminal lumbar interbody fusion with instrumentation. J Neurosurg Spine 2005;3(2): 98–105

24. Patel AA, Zfass-Mendez M, Lebwohl NH, et al. Minimally invasive versus open lumbar fusion: a comparison of blood loss, surgical complications, and hospital course. Iowa Orthop J 2015;35: 130–134

25. Kim MC, Chung HT, Kim DJ, Kim SH, Jeon SH. The clinical and radiological outcomes of minimally invasive transforaminal lumbar interbody single level fusion. Asian Spine J 2011;5(2):111–116

26. Smith ZA, Sugimoto K, Lawton CD, Fessler RG. Incidence of lumbar spine pedicle breach after percutaneous screw fixation: a radiographic evaluation of 601 screws in 151 patients. J Spinal Disord Tech 2014;27(7):358–363

27. Klingler JH, Volz F, Krüger MT, et al. Accidental durotomy in minimally invasive transforaminal lumbar interbody fusion: frequency, risk factors, and management. ScientificWorldJournal 2015; 2015:532628

28. Torres J, James AR, Alimi M, Tsiouris AJ, Geannette C, Härtl R. Screw placement accuracy for minimally invasive transforaminal lumbar interbody fusion surgery: a study on 3-d neuronavigation-guided surgery. Global Spine J 2012;2(3):143–152

29. Wang J, Zhou Y. Perioperative complications related to minimally invasive transforaminal lumbar fusion: evaluation of 204 operations on lumbar instability at single center. Spine J 2014; 14(9):2078–2084

30. Joseph JR, Smith BW, La Marca F, Park P. Comparison of complication rates of minimally invasive transforaminal lumbar interbody fusion and lateral lumbar interbody fusion: a systematic review of the literature. Neurosurg Focus 2015; 39(4):E4

31. Dusad T, Kundnani V, Dutta S, Patel A, Mehta G, Singh M. Comparative prospective study report-ing intraoperative parameters, pedicle screw perforation, and radiation exposure in navigation-guided versus non-navigated fluoroscopy-assisted minimal invasive transforaminal lumbar interbody fusion. Asian Spine J 2018;12(2): 309–316

32. Zhao FD, Yang W, Shan Z, et al. Cage migration after transforaminal lumbar interbody fusion and factors related to it. Orthop Surg 2012;4(4): 227–232

33. Rory J. Petteys, JR, Voyadzis J-M. Two-level minimally invasive transforaminal lumbar inter-body fusion: surgical technique and illustrative cases. ISRN Minim Invasive Surg 2013;201:8

34. Lee WC, Park J-Y, Kim KH, et al. Minimally invasive transforaminal lumbar interbody fusion in multilevel: comparison with conventional trans-foraminal interbody fusion. World Neurosurg 2016;85:236–243

Chapter 5
Endoscopic Transforaminal Lumbar Interbody Fusion

5 Endoscopic Transforaminal Lumbar Interbody Fusion

Sukumar Sura, Said G. Osman, Naresh K. Pagidimarry

Introduction

On the basis of the experiences gained from conventional open and minimally invasive spinal procedures, a long list of desirable objectives has emerged with the evolution of the endoscopic spine surgery. At the top of that list is the desire to minimize the trauma of the surgery and the reductions of surgical blood loss, hospital stay, and complication rates.[1]

Over the past decade, minimally invasive transforaminal lumbar interbody fusion (MIS-TLIF) has become very popular for treating a variety of lumbar spinal disorders. However, MIS-TLIF techniques still require an open incision of the musculature for tube placement. Thus, MIS-TLIF represents an incremental but not revolutionary advancement over the existing open surgical methods.[2]

With the remarkable advancements in endoscopic technologies, the goals of minimally invasive spine surgery including reduced blood loss, less soft tissue destruction, less postoperative pain, and quicker recovery can now be achieved by different surgical endoscopic transforaminal techniques classified according to the properties of the endoscopic system used,[3] that is, percutaneous endoscopic (or full-endoscopic), biportal endoscopic, and microendoscopic.

In this chapter, focus is on the endo-TLIF technique using a working-channel endoscope containing a high-quality optical system and continuous saline irrigation port within the same endoscopic system (single portal) of 6.9 outer diameter.

Indications and Contraindications

Patients who are diagnosed with the following lumbar conditions can benefit from endo-TLIF[4]:

- Lumbar foraminal stenosis with segmental instability.
- Lumbar lateral recess stenosis with segmental instability.
- Lumbar disc herniation with segmental instability.
- Grades 1 and 2 lumbar degenerative/isthmic spondylolisthesis.
- Postoperative instability or failed back surgery syndrome.

Contraindications to endo-TLIF include the following:

- Severe lumbar central stenosis, high-grade spondylolisthesis (grade > 2).
- Severe disc space narrowing.
- Any condition potentially decreasing the safety and effectiveness of a spinal implant, such as osteoporosis, vertebral fracture, infection, or congenital abnormality.

Surgical Methods

Preoperative Planning

The need for meticulous preoperative planning is underscored in any minimally invasive procedure. Careful review of the preoperative radiological studies includes standing lumbar spine anteroposterior and lateral X-rays (flexion and extension); CT and magnetic resonance images (MRI) are essential not only to assess the intended target disc space but also to assess the motion segment.

Careful assessment of the MRI includes evaluating the foramen, lateral recess, and the central canal pathology. Correlation of symptoms with imaging is key.

Measure and record the visual analogue scale scores for low back pain and leg pain, Oswestry disability index, and MacNab criteria preoperatively, for evaluating and comparing with the clinical outcomes postoperatively.

Operative Setup and Anesthesia Techniques

This procedure can be performed with or without general anesthesia. In authors' practice, surgery is performed with epidural analgesia. Use of epidural analgesia reduces the risks associated with general anesthesia and facilitates real-time neurological feedback from the patient. When performed under general anesthesia, it is advisable to perform the procedure while neuromonitoring. The combined effect of epidural anesthesia, least surgical trauma, reduced operating time, and early return to normal activities, allows elderly and patients with co-morbidities to benefit from this procedure.

Surgical Technique

After inducing epidural analgesia and applying sequential compression device for intraoperative deep vein thrombosis prophylaxis, the patient is placed in a prone position on an open-frame radiolucent operating table throughout surgery. Pressure points are checked and padded to protect against injury. Skin preparation is performed with betadine scrub. Draping is done in usual sterile fashion, ensuring wide opening in the drape for the surgical site. The C-arm of the fluoroscope is opposite the surgeon, and the level of the operation is carefully marked on the skin with a sterile felt pen. The skin entry point is identified at the lateral edge of the paravertebral muscle, which typically lays 8 to 13 cm laterally from the midline, depending on the patient's body size.

The procedure starts with injecting local anesthetics into the paravertebral muscle and facet joint and insertion of an 18-gauge, 20-cm spinal needle guided by both anteroposterior and lateral fluoroscopy, to access the disc space transforaminally via Kambin's triangle[5] at the level of interest. Care is taken to ensure the trajectory of the needle is such that the eventual placement of the interbody device is central in anteroposterior view and anterior in the lateral projection. A guide wire is introduced

through the needle, into the disc space, after the removal of stylet. Tapered dilator is advanced over the guide wire and docked into the disc. A bevel-ended 10-mm working cannula is introduced over the dilator. The guidewire and dilator are now withdrawn, and a 4.1-mm working channel endoscope is inserted through the cannula (**Fig. 5.1**) and key anatomical landmarks, including the exiting and traversing nerve roots, were visualized.

Discectomy and end plate preparation for interbody fusion are performed using a combination of pituitary forceps, reamer, curettes, osteotomes, and bipolar radiofrequency under fluoroscopic and endoscopic visualization. The reamer is expanded within the disc space and rotated back and forth in the disc space to excise the disc material and fibrocartilage from the end plates. Endoscopic visualization ensures the adequacy of end plate preparation. The adequacy of end plate preparation is confirmed by visualization of the subchondral bone and petechial bleeding as shown in **Fig. 5.2**. Care is taken to preserve the subchondral bone to minimize the risk of subsidence of interbody cage.

Following end plate preparation, morselized allograft mixed with bone marrow aspirate, obtained from the iliac crest (**Fig. 5.3**) or autogenous cancellous bone graft is inserted anteriorly into the disc space through working cannula (**Fig. 5.4**).

Once the fusion site preparation is done, endoscopic system is withdrawn, and the interbody fusion cage is delivered through the working cannula using a cage delivery tool under fluoroscopic guidance (**Fig. 5.5**).

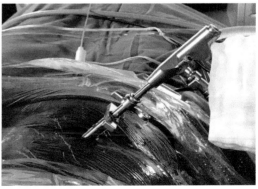

Fig. 5.1 Working channel endoscope is inserted through working cannula.

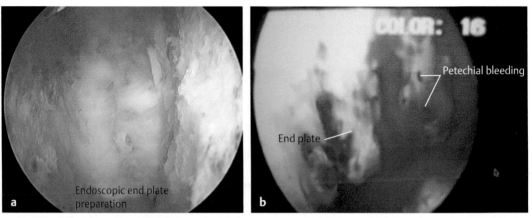

Fig. 5.2 (a, b) Endoscopic visualization of end plate preparation.

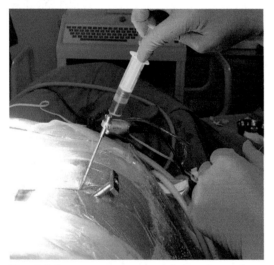

Fig. 5.3 Bone marrow aspirate being drawn from the iliac crest.

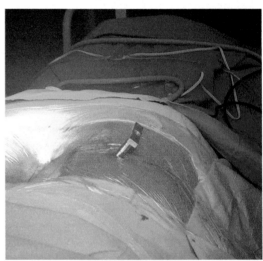

Fig. 5.4 Working cannula in situ.

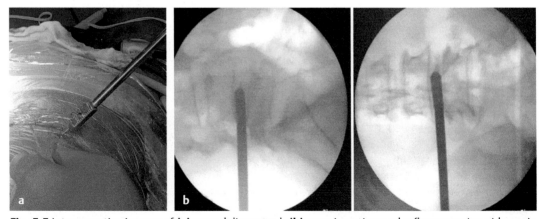

Fig. 5.5 Intraoperative images of **(a)** cage delivery tool, **(b)** cage insertion under fluoroscopic guidance in both anteroposterior and lateral view.

Pedicle screws or facet screws are placed after cage insertion. Using Jamshidi needle, pedicles are entered percutaneously under fluoroscopic guidance. Guidewire is placed through Jamshidi needle. Serial dilators are passed over the guidewire. Pedicle screw system is inserted over the guidewire and rod placement is done as per the system used (**Fig. 5.6**).

Clinical Outcomes and Complications

It is now about 16 years since the first documented case of endoscopic transforaminal lumbar decompression and interbody fusion was performed.[1] Over this period of time,

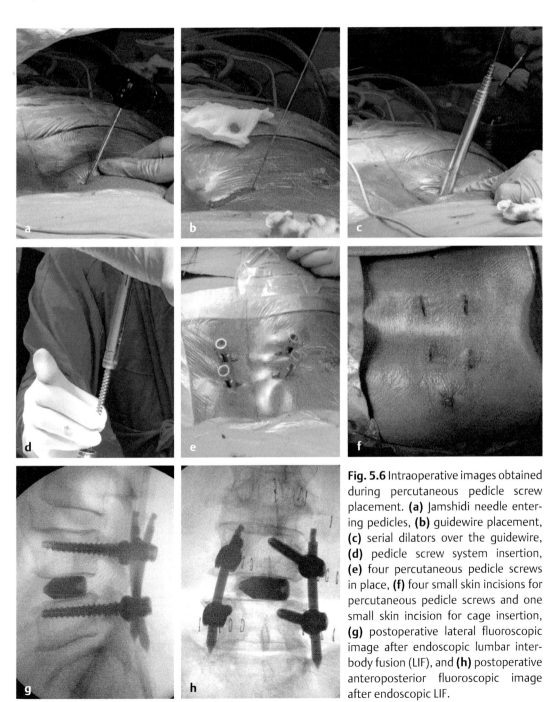

Fig. 5.6 Intraoperative images obtained during percutaneous pedicle screw placement. **(a)** Jamshidi needle entering pedicles, **(b)** guidewire placement, **(c)** serial dilators over the guidewire, **(d)** pedicle screw system insertion, **(e)** four percutaneous pedicle screws in place, **(f)** four small skin incisions for percutaneous pedicle screws and one small skin incision for cage insertion, **(g)** postoperative lateral fluoroscopic image after endoscopic lumbar interbody fusion (LIF), and **(h)** postoperative anteroposterior fluoroscopic image after endoscopic LIF.

technological evolution and experience with the approach have consistently produced least amount of surgical trauma, minimal collateral damage, reduced surgical time, reduced hospital stay, reduced risk of complications, short rehabilitation, early return to productive life, and reduced cost of care.

Intraoperative complications, such as end plate fracture and suboptimal positioning of cage, are possible. Nerve root injury can happen during cage insertion; more commonly, postoperative dysesthesia is seen following transforaminal instrumentation. In general, the dysesthesia settles within 3 weeks postoperatively, in the majority of cases.

Advantages over TLIF Techniques

The following are the key advantages of endo-TLIF over open fusion surgery or MIS-TLIF:

- Significantly less operating time.
- Less stress for the operating team.
- Better endoscopic visualization of the adequacy of neural decompression and end plate preparation.
- Procedure can be performed under epidural analgesia.
- Least amount of trauma to paraspinal muscles and preservation of bony structure.
- Minimal blood loss with virtually no need for transfusion.
- Minimal risk of intra- or postoperative complications.
- Outpatient of short hospital stay.
- Short duration of the use of opioid medication.

- Short rehabilitation program.
- Early return to productive life.
- High medium- and long-term success rate.

Conclusion

Endo-TLIF in its true form is the least invasive procedure among all the approaches in lumbar interbody fusion. The key concept and early results of endo-TLIF are promising; however, the surgical technique requires a complex and time consuming learning curve especially in those who are not trained in endoscopic techniques.

References

1. Osman SG. Endoscopic transforaminal decompression, interbody fusion, and percutaneous pedicle screw implantation of the lumbar spine: a case series report. Int J Spine Surg 2012;6: 157–166
2. Kolcun JPG, Brusko GD, Basil GW, Epstein R, Wang MY. Endoscopic transforaminal lumbar interbody fusion without general anesthesia: operative and clinical outcomes in 100 consecutive patients with a minimum 1-year follow-up. Neurosurg Focus 2019;46(4):E14
3. Birkenmaier C, Komp M, Leu HF, Wegener B, Ruetten S. The current state of endoscopic disc surgery: review of controlled studies comparing full-endoscopic procedures for disc herniations to standard procedures. Pain Physician 2013; 16(4):335–344
4. Ahn Y, Youn MS, Heo DH. Endoscopic transforaminal lumbar interbody fusion: a comprehensive review. Expert Rev Med Devices 2019; 16(5):373–380
5. Kambin P. Arthroscopic microdiscectomy. Arthroscopy 1992;8(3):287–295

Chapter 6
Posterior Lumbar Interbody Fusion

6 Posterior Lumbar Interbody Fusion

J. K. B. C. Parthiban

Introduction

Posterior lumbar interbody fusion (PLIF) was first described by Briggs and Milligan in 1944[1] and further modifications to the procedure with surgical descriptions were made by Jaslow in 1946[2] and Cloward in 1953.[3] Briggs used bone chips from local laminectomy as interbody graft and Jaslow used spinous processes. However, the technique of PLIF was made popular by Cloward who introduced iliac autografts. This technique yielded better fusion rates (>85%) compared with any other previous PLIF technique or posterolateral fusions (PLFs).[4] In PLIF, disc removal and end plate preparation are carried out medial to the facet joint with retraction of the dura and nerve roots. This dural retraction in untrained hands resulted in complications such as dural injuries, graft extrusion, arachnoiditis, etc. and hence it did not gain expected popularity until 1990s. The introduction of interbody instrumentation and implants had made PLIF easy to perform and it also gained a wide reach since then.[5] Though, several approaches are available for performing interbody fusion, the entire principle was derived from PLIF and this technique is still routinely performed by many surgeons.

Indications

The indications for PLIF include unstable spinal pathologies, such as spondylolisthesis, degenerative lumbar scoliosis, and lumbar canal stenosis, which require adequate stabilization. PLIF procedure is ideally recommended for patients with neurogenic claudication secondary to significant ligamentum flavum hypertrophy with relatively normal facets. The extended indications are recurrent disc prolapse, spondylodiscitis, back pain secondary to degenerative disc diseases and failed fusions. This procedure is preferably done at L4–L5, L5–S1 spinal pathologies for easier retraction of cauda equina roots without injury.

Preoperative Planning

Patients having lumbar spine pathology with relatively normal facets are good candidates for performing PLIF without facetectomy. However, in the presence of facet-hypertrophy-related radicular pain, facetectomy is unavoidable. Dynamic radiographs in standing position are good to identify spine instability (**Fig. 6.1**) which may not be picked up by routine

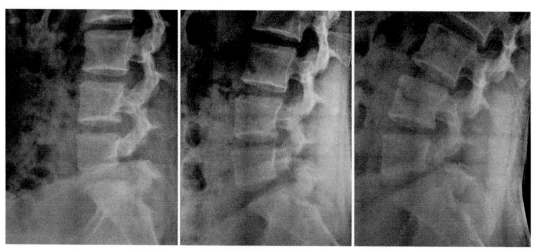

Fig. 6.1 Dynamic radiograph demonstrating instability and pars lysis.

magnetic resonance imaging (MRI). The whole-spine radiograph along with hip joints help in the measurement of pelvic parameters, lumbar lordosis, thoracic kyphosis, thereby aiding in the assessment of spinal balance. Computed tomography scan can help in assessing pedicle size and trajectory, detect any lysis in pars interarticularis, especially for conditions such as dysplastic spondylolisthesis. Adjacent level disc and facet joint morphology assessment by MRI helps in deciding the level of fusion. Rare instances of neural anomalies like conjoined nerve roots that can preclude PLIF procedure can be identified by MRI.

Surgical Steps

The PLIF procedure consists of four sequential steps that are as follows:

1. Exposure and pedicle screw insertion.
2. Decompression and exposure of PLIF corridor.
3. Discectomy and end plate preparation.
4. Interbody grafting and cage insertion.

Exposure and Pedicle Screw Insertion

The patient is positioned prone following intubation and two bolsters are placed under to accentuate lordosis. If iliac crest harvesting is planned, the exact site should be marked and prepared. A midline incision is made, and the para spinal muscles are separated from spinolaminar surface laterally to expose the facet joints and base of the transverse process at the required level. Electrocautery helps in exposure and also provides hemostasis; however, few surgeons may prefer sharp dissection by scalpel. Careful attention should be paid not to damage the joint capsule of the cranial motion segment while using electrocautery. This is the key to avoid adjacent segment degeneration. This exposure also gives adequate space for posterolateral grafting when required and for good pedicle preparation to insert the pedicle screws. A thorough and neat dissection of the lamina, facet joints, and interlaminar space is a prerequisite for proper orientation to the PLIF corridor (**Fig. 6.2**).

Decompression and Exposure of PLIF Corridor

The interspinous ligaments are removed with rongeurs to expose the interlaminar space. During this process, inferior half of the spinous process is removed preserving the superior half to maintain the posterior ligamentous complex of adjacent motion segment. In the present era, high-speed drill and 45-degree Kerrison punches are used to create the corridor.

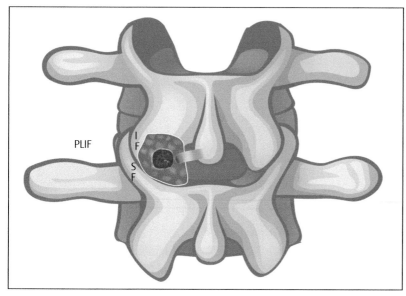

Fig. 6.2 Schema of posterior lumbar interbody fusion corridor. PLIF, posterior lumbar interbody fusion.

This is in contrast to chisels and hammers used previously; however, utilizing drills has to be kept minimum as it might result in loss of local bone grafts. The ligamentum flavum is then removed in a usual fashion from cranial to caudal end without damaging the dura. In case of a mild facet hypertrophy, removal of inferior facets may not be needed. At times, surgeons prefer to trim the medial third of inferior facet for easy retraction. When the facet is significantly hypertrophied, the inferior part of the superior lamina along with the inferior facet of the upper vertebra is excised, exposing the articulating surface of the superior facet of lower vertebra (**Fig. 6.3**). The medial one-third of the superior facet can be trimmed further to decompress the lateral recess adequately (**Figs. 6.4 and 6.5**). Subsequently, the superior rim of inferior lamina is excised up till

reaching the pedicle laterally. Care should be taken while performing this step, as the ligamentum flavum is attached to the rim and the dura is adjacent within the spinal canal at this level (**Fig. 6.6**). The same steps are completed on the opposite side.

Once the ligamentum flavum is excised all around (**Fig. 6.7**), the PLIF corridor can be visualized containing the dura, dural sleeve of descending nerve root, lateral dural margin, epidural plexus over the lateral part of annulus, and posterior surface of the vertebral body (**Fig. 6.8**). The visualized epidural veins within the corridor need to be cleared from the dural margin for approaching the intervertebral space. Epidural venous bleed is controlled with microtip bipolar low cautery, hemostats, and cottonoids (**Fig. 6.9**) and then cut with microscissors (**Fig. 6.10**). The dura and nerve root are

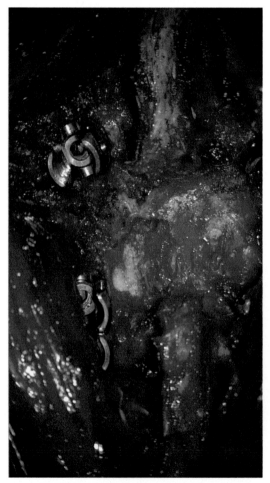

Fig. 6.3 Inferior facetectomy of superior vertebra done.

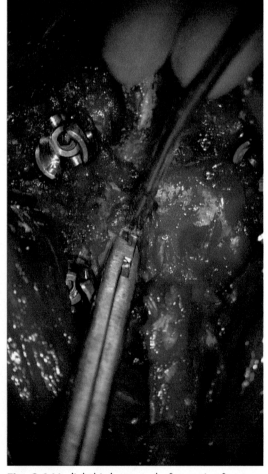

Fig. 6.4 Medial third removal of superior facet on process.

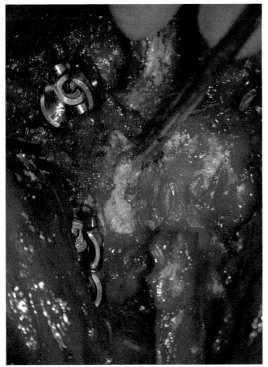

Fig. 6.5 Articulating surface of superior facet seen with medial third removed.

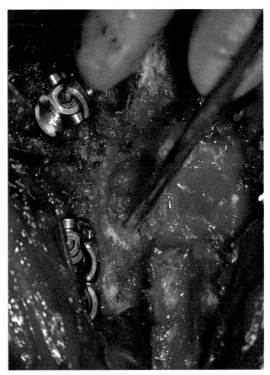

Fig. 6.6 Superior rim of inferior lamina removed with rongeur carefully.

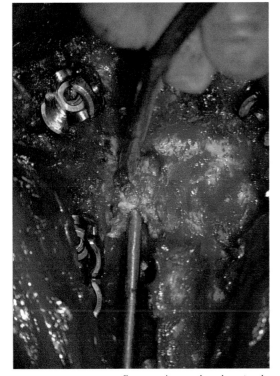

Fig. 6.7 Ligamentum flavum elevated and excised.

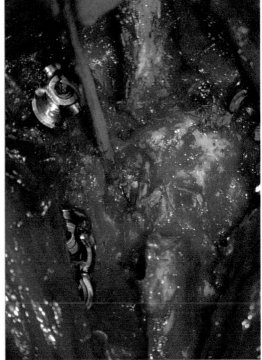

Fig. 6.8 Visualization of dura, nerve root, lateral part of disc annulus, and epidural veins after flavectomy.

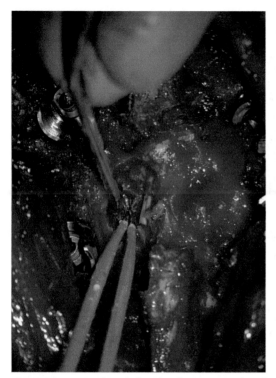

Fig. 6.9 Batson's plexus of epidural veins coagulated with bipolar cautery.

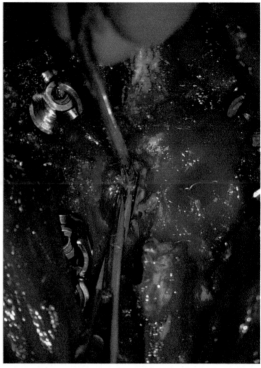

Fig. 6.10 Cutting of coagulated veins using microscissors.

gently retracted and placed medially with the help of nerve root retractor. This can be held in place by inserting cottonoids in the epidural spaces above and below (**Fig. 6.11**). This technique is quite old fashioned, but very effective in keeping the nerve root away and protected. The area present lateral to the dura and medial to the trimmed facets/laminar edges exposes lateral annular surface of disc for further procedure. Decompression of the opposite lateral recess can be done by deroofing and extending the laminectomy to the opposite side (**Fig. 6.12**).

Discectomy and End Plate Preparation

The annulus is cut vertically lateral to the dural border and horizontally at the edges of the margin of vertebral body as far as possible and removed as a single piece of cake (**Fig. 6.13**). This window in the annulus is the main entry point to the disc space. It is advised not to retract the dura across the midline to avoid traction injury to the nerve, particularly at the level of L4–L5 or higher. The window may be pretty

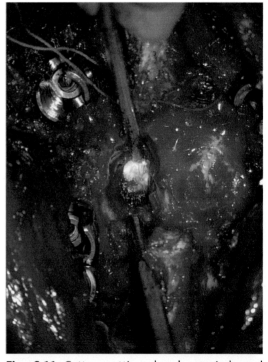

Fig. 6.11 Cotton patties placed superiorly and inferiorly to retract the nerve root and expose the annulus.

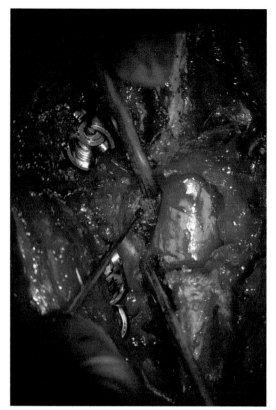

Fig. 6.12 Laminectomy and deroofing of opposite lateral recess.

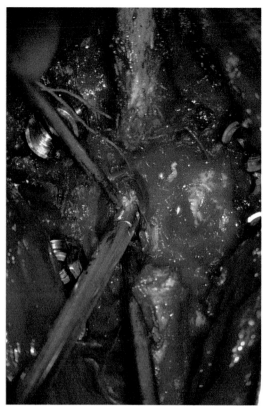

Fig. 6.13 Annulotomy and discectomy.

small in patients with severe stenosis and/or listhesis. The posterior superior rim of vertebral body can be chiseled from posterior through the cartilage rim and into the disc space. This is to enhance the window and at the lateral aspect, it can be as close to pedicle as possible. Degenerated disc material can be removed in pieces from the entire disc space using round-tipped disc-grasping forceps. Forward angulated forceps can also be used to remove the disc material from far lateral side. Surgeon can feel the anterior border of the intervertebral space and care should be taken never to use force while doing so since it is slippery. The central part is wide giving way when a forceful insertion of the forceps is attempted toward the anterior border. Accidental penetration of anterior annulus and anterior longitudinal ligament can be disastrous.

The cartilaginous end plate on the adjoining vertebral bodies within the disc space is later scooped and scraped away from the cortex at the side of the corridor (**Fig. 6.14a and b**) and then at the far end (**Fig. 6.14c and d**) using different curettes containing rugged edges. End plate preparation is then performed with sequential increase in the size of the reamers, small osteotomes, and curved sharp instrument to facilitate a fertile surface for bone grafting. Once these steps are followed, the intervertebral disc space is now ready for bone grafting. The same procedure is repeated on the other side as well, especially when bilateral cage insertion is planned.

Interbody Grafting and Cage Insertion

In LIF, the biological part of fusion is provided by the local morselized spinolaminar grafts or iliac grafts (classic PLIF). If local corticocancellous bone grafts are planned to be used, they are packed tight for few millimeters from anterior to posterior vertebrae to prevent any graft extrusions into canal and impacted (**Fig. 6.15a–c**). There are various described techniques of bone

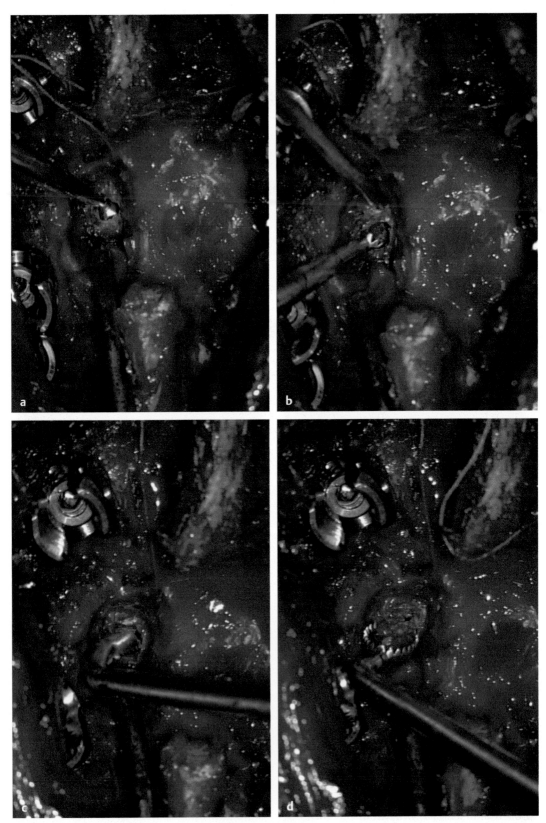

Fig. 6.14 (a–d) End plate preparation by different curettes.

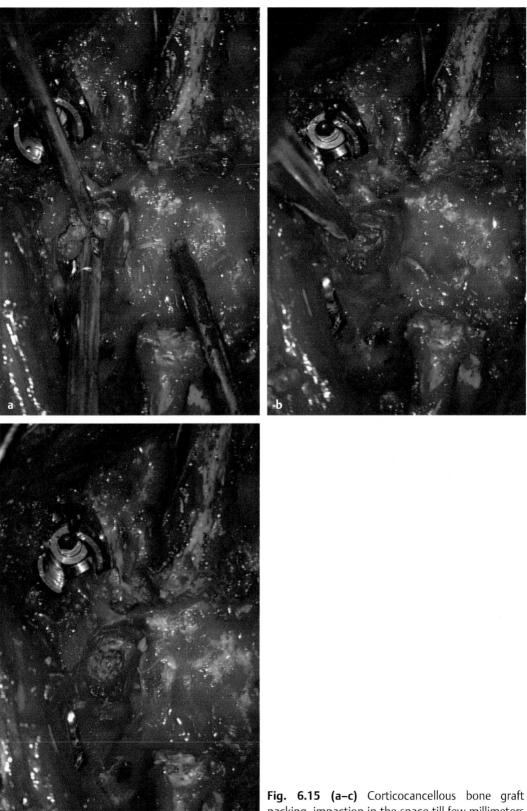

Fig. 6.15 (a–c) Corticocancellous bone graft packing, impaction in the space till few millimeters anterior to canal.

graft placements adapted by different authors (**Fig. 6.16**). The advantage of using local bone grafts is avoiding the morbidity of the grafts site. In classic PLIF, tricortical and bicortical bones harvested from posterior iliac crest are inserted in the disc space as shown (**Fig. 6.17**).

Interbody rigid implants are commonly used in addition to grafts to achieve mechanical stability and indirect decompression of exiting roots, and to maintain the disc height and carry out sagittal correction. The cage implants act as mechanical supports to prevent settling of intervertebral space by providing support to anterior column and pedicle screws (**Fig. 6.18**). The various cages available over few decades include Bagby and Kuslich (BAK) cylindrical perforated stainless steel cages, Brantigan carbon fiber-reinforced polymer (CFRP) cages, titanium, and polyether ether ketone (PEEK) cages. These cages are usually inserted along with bone grafts. The choice of interbody implant for PLIF is bullet-shaped PEEK cages that are inserted almost vertically with minimal

medial angulation into the prepared disc space bilaterally. These cages are filled with locally harvested cancellous bones in the anterior part of disc space after an initial distraction achieved through the pedicle screws (**Fig. 6.19**). Since PLIF corridor is narrower than TLIF, the width of the cages must be relatively smaller making bullet-shaped cages the preferable choice. The PLIF construct is completed with application of rods on to the pedicle screws (**Fig. 6.20**) with mild compression on the PLIF cage to maintain lumbar lordosis (**Fig. 6.21**).

When a scenario such as limitation of disc space/nerve root anomalies blocking the access to the space/limited ability to retract nerve roots (secondary to epidural scarring) arises, a unilateral cage can be placed achieving results similar to bilateral cages.[6] Various studies have proven that a unilateral cage can be as stable and stiff as bilateral cages. The cage position does not affect the stability of the construct and they are more stable with bilateral pedicle screw fixation.[7-13] It is recommended that 77% of

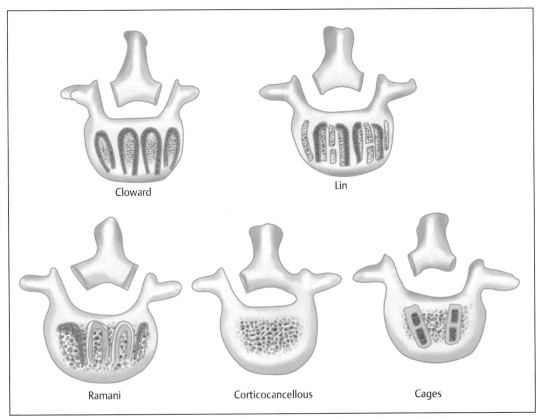

Fig. 6.16 Different bone grafting techniques adapted in posterior lumbar interbody fusion.

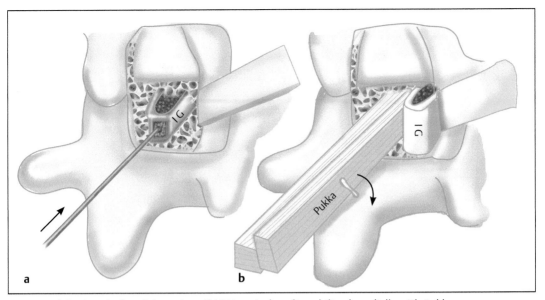

Fig. 6.17 (a) Tricortical graft insertion. **(b)** Tricortical graft mobilized medially with Pukka.

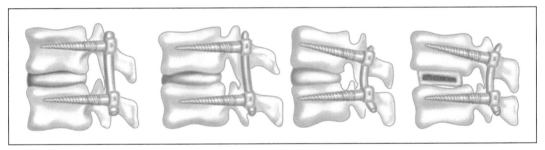

Fig. 6.18 Role of cage in posterior lumbar interbody fusion construct—prevents settling of disc space by giving anterior support.

available disc space should be packed with bone grafts for a successful fusion. Hence, bone grafts in addition needs to be inserted before the cage insertion.[14] Closkey et al found that > 30% of the vertebral end plate surface is required for load transmission across structural interbody grafts by in vitro analysis.[15]

Outcomes and Complications

The clinical and radiological outcomes of PLIF are influenced by various factors such as skill of the surgeon, end plate preparation, type of cage and grafts used, adequacy of decompression, instrumentation, and the most important being proper patient selection. A meta-analysis of nine studies comparing PLF and PLIF for isthmic spondylolisthesis revealed lower fusion rates in PLF ($p = 0.005$, odds ratio [OR] = 0.29 [0.14, 0.58]).[16] The fusion rates in PLIF vary from as low as 72%[17] to as high as 95%[18-21] regardless of the cage used. This reinstates that the key factor for fusion is adequate end plate preparation. The iliac grafts are excellent material for fusion but graft site morbidity is reported to be 25%.[22] In scenarios where two-level PLIF is done, 85% had complete fusion and the nonunion is mainly at the caudal level (predominantly L5–S1).[23] One study has demonstrated good fusion rates without loss of sagittal balance even when stand-alone local bone grafts are used for single-level fusion.[24] A study has shown better clinical outcomes by demonstrating significant

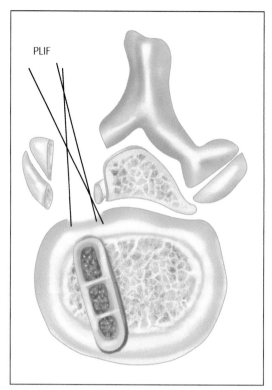

Fig. 6.19 Cage insertion into anterior part of disc space. PLIF, posterior lumbar interbody fusion.

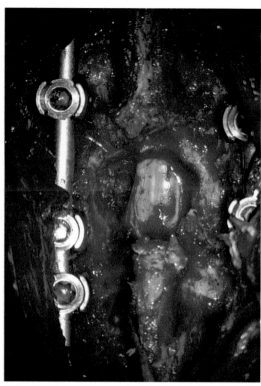

Fig. 6.20 Completion of posterior lumbar interbody fusion construct by rods insertion.

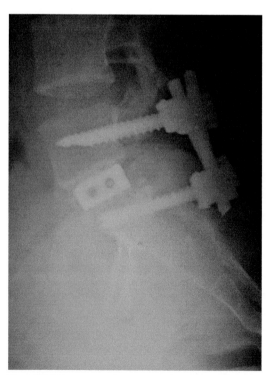

Fig. 6.21 Postoperative X-ray of posterior lumbar interbody fusion construct with good lordosis.

improvement of modified Japanese Orthopaedic Association score from 10.8 to 19.6 with mean recovery rate being 47.7%.[25]

The most common complication which led to replacement of PLIF by TLIF is the inadvertent chance of nerve root injuries producing foot drop when operated at L4–L5 levels. The reported complication rates vary from 0.4 to 13.6%.[26,27] These nerve root injuries can be avoided by wider resection of facets, adequate decompression, and selection of an appropriate cage with careful retraction of the nerve roots. The other complications such as graft displacement, cage backouts, subsidence, pseudoarthrosis, dural injuries, which are common in any LIF procedure can also be present in PLIF.[28]

Conclusion

PLIF is technically challenging and is the precursor of all LIF techniques. It provides adequate anterior support and good fusion without an anterior incision. Adequate visualization of the

PLIF corridor, careful retraction of the dural tube, and avoidance of oversized cages are essential learning steps for a successful surgery and better postoperative outcome.

Tips and Tricks

- PLIF is best at L5–S1 level, as the interlaminar space is wider at this level. It can be done bilaterally at L5–S1, L4–L5 at ease.

- When approached from one side, it can be applied at all levels, provided corticocancellous bones alone are used for grafting.

- Dural and sleeve retraction may lead to nerve root damage and in particular at L4–L5 and higher levels. This can be avoided by doing bilateral wide facetectomy for easy retraction and using adequate-sized cage.

- Some surgeons prefer to preserve the dorsal one-third of the interspinous ligament to maintain the tension band and limit the extensive retraction of nerve roots.[4]

- Cages that cannot be placed medially at the midline/angulated medially can be managed by using corticocancellous bone grafts alone (**Fig. 6.22**).

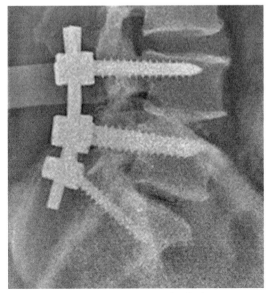

Fig. 6.22 Posterior lumbar interbody fusion L4–L5 with spinolaminar corticocancellous bone grafts.

References

1. Briggs H, Milligan P. Chip fusion of the low back following exploration of the spinal canal. J Bone Joint Surg. 1944;26:125–130

2. Jaslow IA. Intercorporal bone graft in spinal fusion after disc removal. Surg Gynecol Obstet 1946;82:215–218

3. Cloward RB. The treatment of ruptured lumbar intervertebral discs by vertebral body fusion. I. Indications, operative technique, after care. J Neurosurg 1953;10(2):154–168

4. Cole CD, McCall TD, Schmidt MH, Dailey AT. Comparison of low back fusion techniques: transforaminal lumbar interbody fusion (TLIF) or posterior lumbar interbody fusion (PLIF) approaches. Curr Rev Musculoskelet Med 2009; 2(2):118–126

5. Turner JA, Ersek M, Herron L, et al. Patient outcomes after lumbar spinal fusions. JAMA 1992;268(7):907–911

6. Fogel GR, Toohey JS, Neidre A, Brantigan JW. Is one cage enough in posterior lumbar interbody fusion: a comparison of unilateral single cage interbody fusion to bilateral cages. J Spinal Disord Tech 2007;20(1):60–65

7. Ames CP, Acosta FL Jr, Chi J, et al. Biomechanical comparison of posterior lumbar interbody fusion and transforaminal lumbar interbody fusion performed at 1 and 2 levels. Spine 2005;30(19): E562–E566

8. Chen HH, Cheung HH, Wang WK, Li A, Li KC. Biomechanical analysis of unilateral fixation with interbody cages. Spine 2005;30(4):E92–E96

9. Kettler A, Schmoelz W, Kast E, Gottwald M, Claes L, Wilke HJ. In vitro stabilizing effect of a transforaminal compared with two posterior lumbar interbody fusion cages. Spine 2005;30(22): E665–E670

10. Harris BM, Hilibrand AS, Savas PE, et al. Transforaminal lumbar interbody fusion: the effect of various instrumentation techniques on the flexibility of the lumbar spine. Spine 2004; 29(4):E65–E70

11. Heth JA, Hitchon PW, Goel VK, Rogge TN, Drake JS, Torner JC. A biomechanical comparison between anterior and transverse interbody fusion cages. Spine 2001;26(12):E261–E267

12. Wang ST, Goel VK, Fu CY, et al. Posterior instrumentation reduces differences in spine stability as a result of different cage orientations: an in vitro study. Spine 2005;30(1):62–67

13. Javernick MA, Kuklo TR, Polly DW Jr. Transforaminal lumbar interbody fusion: unilateral versus bilateral disk removal—an in vivo study. Am J Orthop 2003;32(7):344–348, discussion 348

14. Prolo DJ, Oklund SA, Butcher M. Toward uniformity in evaluating results of lumbar spine

operations. A paradigm applied to posterior lumbar interbody fusions. Spine 1986;11(6): 601–606

15. Closkey RF, Parsons JR, Lee CK, Blacksin MF, Zimmerman MC. Mechanics of interbody spinal fusion. Analysis of critical bone graft area. Spine 1993;18(8):1011–1015

16. Luo J, Cao K, Yu T, et al. Comparison of posterior lumbar interbody fusion versus posterolateral fusion for the treatment of isthmic spondylolisthesis. Clin Spine Surg 2017;30(7): E915–E922

17. Fuji T, Oda T, Kato Y, Fujita S, Tanaka M. Posterior lumbar interbody fusion using titanium cylindrical threaded cages: is optimal interbody fusion possible without other instrumentation? J Orthop Sci 2003;8(2):142–147

18. Brantigan JW, Steffee AD, Lewis ML, Quinn LM, Persenaire JM. Lumbar interbody fusion using the Brantigan I/F cage for posterior lumbar interbody fusion and the variable pedicle screw placement system: two-year results from a Food and Drug Administration investigational device exemption clinical trial. Spine 2000;25(11):1437–1446

19. Arnold PM, Robbins S, Paullus W, Faust S, Holt R, McGuire R. Clinical outcomes of lumbar degenerative disc disease treated with posterior lumbar interbody fusion allograft spacer: a prospective, multicenter trial with 2-year follow-up. Am J Orthop 2009;38(7):E115–E122

20. Kuslich SD, Danielson G, Dowdle JD, et al. Four-year follow-up results of lumbar spine arthrodesis using the Bagby and Kuslich lumbar fusion cage. Spine 2000;25(20):2656–2662

21. Manabe H, Sakai T, Morimoto M, et al. Radiological outcomes of posterior lumbar interbody fusion using a titanium-coated PEEK cage. J Med Invest 2019;66(1.2):119–122

22. Gibson S, McLeod I, Wardlaw D, Urbaniak S. Allograft versus autograft in instrumented posterolateral lumbar spinal fusion: a randomized control trial. Spine 2002;27(15):1599–1603

23. Aono H, Takenaka S, Nagamoto Y, et al. Fusion rate and clinical outcomes in two-level posterior lumbar interbody fusion. World Neurosurg 2018; 112:e473–e478

24. Govindasamy R, Solomon P, Sugumar D, Gnanadoss JJ, Murugan Y, Najimudeen S. Is the cage an additional hardware in lumbar interbody fusion for low grade spondylolisthesis? a prospective study. J Clin Diagn Res 2017;11(5):RC05–RC08

25. Takahashi Y, Okuda S, Nagamoto Y, Matsumoto T, Sugiura T, Iwasaki M. Effect of segmental lordosis on the clinical outcomes of 2-level posterior lumbar interbody fusion for 2-level degenerative lumbar spondylolisthesis. J Neurosurg Spine 2019;1–6. doi: 10.3171/2019.4.SPINE181463. [Epub ahead of print].

26. Davne SH, Myers DL. Complications of lumbar spinal fusion with transpedicular instrumentation. Spine 1992;17(6, Suppl):S184–S189

27. Barnes B, Rodts GE Jr, Haid RW Jr, Subach BR, McLaughlin MR. Allograft implants for posterior lumbar interbody fusion: results comparing cylindrical dowels and impacted wedges. Neurosurgery 2002;51(5):1191–1198, discussion 1198

28. Okuda S, Miyauchi A, Oda T, Haku T, Yamamoto T, Iwasaki M. Surgical complications of posterior lumbar interbody fusion with total facetectomy in 251 patients. J Neurosurg Spine 2006;4(4): 304–309

Chapter 7

Lateral Interbody Fusion: Extreme Lateral Interbody Fusion/Direct Lateral Interbody Fusion

7 Lateral Interbody Fusion: Extreme Lateral Interbody Fusion/Direct Lateral Interbody Fusion

Yong Hai, Peng Yin, Yaoshen Zhang, Yiqi Zhang

Introduction

The incidence rate of lumbar spine fusion for the treatment of various degenerative lumbar spine diseases has increased significantly over the past 20 years.[1] A variety of lumbar spine fusion techniques have been developed and popularized, such as anterior lumbar interbody fusion (ALIF), posterior lumbar interbody fusion (PLIF), transforaminal lumbar interbody fusion (TLIF), and lateral lumbar interbody fusion (LLIF). Traditional open spinal surgery could acquire a satisfactory effect, but extensive destruction of muscle and ligaments usually leads to tremendous postoperative pain, muscular atrophy, and functional disability. Recently, extreme lateral interbody fusion (XLIF)/direct lateral interbody fusion (DLIF) has been introduced for the spine fusion due to the advantage of the characteristics of minimally invasive surgery. XLIF (NuVasive, San Diego, CA) and DLIF (Medtronic, Memphis, TN) belong to the same type of surgery in essence, and the reason for different denomination is the difference of surgical instruments by the two companies. XLIF takes advantage of a unique surgical corridor to the spinal column; therefore, the fusion technique could afford maximal disc excision, end plate availability, and indirect decompression of the neural elements. Ozgur et al first described XLIF in 2006[2]; the technique could identify a safe corridor for exposure due to the advances in neuromonitoring during the operation. XLIF is achieved via a minimally invasive lateral, retroperitoneal, transpsoas approach to access the targeted disc space. The chapter summarizes the preoperative planning, indications and contradictions, operative technique, clinical results, and complications of XLIF.

Indications and Contraindications

Indications for the XLIF technique are most suitable for interbody access from L2–4. The patients typically suffer degenerative disc disease with or without instability, discogenic pain due to segmental instability, lumbar spinal stenosis (LSS), degenerative scoliosis, adjacent segmental disease, and degenerative spondylolisthesis (grade I or II).[3–5] XLIF could be operated at L1–2 intervertebral space, but demands either removal or maneuvering around the descending twentieth rib. The technique could also be performed at L4–5 intervertebral space; however, there will be a higher risk of nerve root injury. In addition, the height of iliac crests should be confirmed whether L4–5 can be accessed directly or not. The relative contradictions include L5–S1 level, degenerative spondylolisthesis (grade III or IV), severe degenerative scoliosis, and bilateral retroperitoneal scarring. Also, the XLIF technique can be combined with staged posterior decompression and fixation or posterior–lateral fusion if necessary.

Preoperative Planning

Detailed preoperative planning plays a key role in performing a successful XLIF surgery; hence, authors suggest meticulous preoperative medical and cardiovascular evaluations. Furthermore, sufficient radiological evaluation is conducive to avoiding potential problems on the surgical approach. For instance, at upper levels (L1–2), confirmation of rib location facilitates prevention of any unexpected conditions during the operation. At lower levels (L4–5), the height of the iliac crest should be examined to ensure there will be clearance into the disc space.

Operative Technique

Patient Preparation

The patient with the XLIF technique receives general anesthesia, and then the patient is placed on a bendable surgical table in a true 90-degree lateral decubitus position (**Fig. 7.1**). The patient is secured laterally with tape to ensure that the pelvis tilts away from the spine, allowing access to all the lumbar levels, especially L4–5. With the help of fluoroscopy, the targeted level is confirmed, and the surgical table should be flexed in proper extent to increase the distance from the iliac crest to the ribs to gain direct access to the disc. If the patient is diagnosed with degenerative scoliosis, authors prefer to approach from the concavity side.

Incision and Retroperitoneal Access

After aseptic treatment of the operative skin region, two Kirschner wires (K-wire) are employed to identify the mid position of the disc of interest with the assistance of fluoroscopy (**Fig. 7.2**). One line is drawn over the center of the targeted disc in an anteroposterior direction. Another line is drawn though the center of the neighboring vertebral bodies in a superoinferior direction. A small skin incision is made where these lines cross for inserting the atraumatic tissue dilators and an expandable retractor, which will be the working portal. An incision is made posterolaterally to introduce an index finger into the retroperitoneal space to sweep open the space. At this step, the layers of the lateral abdominal muscles (external oblique, internal oblique, transversus, and the transversal fascia) should be identified and opened one by one until the retroperitoneal fat is reached. The main goal of the step is to ensure that all lateral attachments of the peritoneum are released to provide safe lateral entry (**Fig. 7.3**).

Transpsoas Access

After the retroperitoneal space is identified, the index finger is brought up under the lateral skin, and an incision is created at this direct location for the insertion of an initial dilator. The finger is applied in the retroperitoneal space to guide the dilator safely from the incision to the psoas muscle (**Fig. 7.4**). The dilator is then placed over the surface of the psoas muscle, accurately over the targeted disc space, identified by fluoroscopy. The fibers of the psoas muscle are gently dissected with the dilators until the disc of interest is reached. The electromyography monitoring system is employed to assess the proximity of the lumbar nerve roots to the advancing dilator (**Fig. 7.5**). An expandable retractor is used over the last dilator (**Fig. 7.6**).

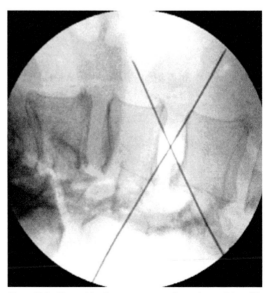

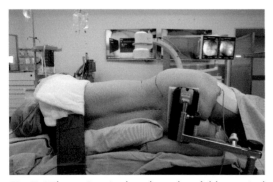

Fig. 7.1 The patient is placed on a bendable surgical table in a true 90-degree lateral decubitus position. The position is used to elevate and elongate the space between the ribs and iliac crest.

Fig. 7.2 Two K-wires are employed to identify the midposition of the disc of interest with the assistance of fluoroscopy.

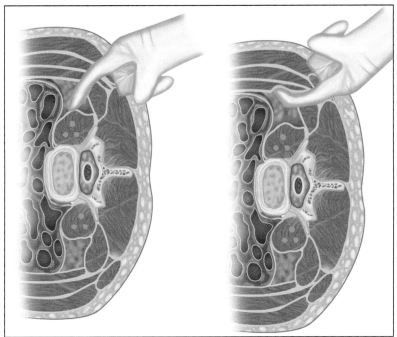

Fig. 7.3 The index finger is used to perform retroperitoneal dissection. Blunt approach is made to the retroperitoneal space through the layers of the lateral abdominal muscles. The finger is inserted into the retroperitoneal space to sweep open. The finger should be used to widen the space both deep and backwards to the incision site.

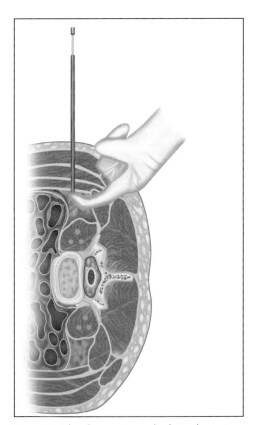

Fig. 7.4 The finger is applied in the retroperitoneal space to guide the initial dilation safely from the incision to the psoas muscle.

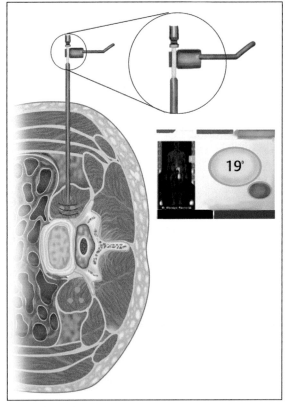

Fig. 7.5 The electromyography monitoring system is employed to assess the proximity of the lumbar nerve roots to the advancing dilator.

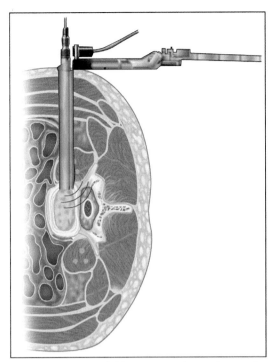

Fig. 7.6 An expandable retractor is used over the last dilator.

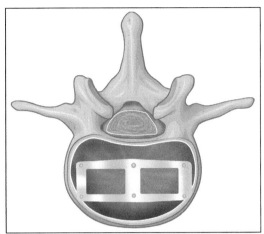

Fig. 7.7 The extreme lateral interbody fusion cage spans the ring apophysis to provide the maximum vertebral support.

Preparing the Disc and Device Implantation

Under direct-illuminated vision, the step is performed as a conventional open surgery: disc removal, end plate preparation, and implant insertion. First, a thorough discectomy is performed. The annulotomy is created at least 18-mm long in an anteroposterior direction. The annulotomy window should be centered in the anterior lateral half of the disc space of interest. Disc removal and release of the contralateral annulus were made by a Cobb elevator to obtain the opportunity to place a long implant cage. Pituitary rongeurs, curettes, disc cutters, scrapers, and other related instruments are used to evacuate the disc and prepare the end plates for fusion. After the completion of disc preparation, the XLIF cage with mixture of autogenous and artificial bone grafts is introduced from a lateral direction into the targeted disc space. The cage should be placed on both lateral margins of the apophyseal ring to maximize end plate support, restore intervertebral height, and correct

imbalance alignment (**Fig. 7.7**). The internal fixations would be performed or not depending on patient's specific conditions.

Closure

The expandable retractor is collapsed and removed slowly to allow the surgeon to observe the psoas muscle and confirm hemostasis. The incision is sutured layer by layer.

Cases

Lumbar spinal stenosis is an indication for XLIF technique. A 66-year-old male patient suffered from low back pain for 40 years and progressed for 3 months. He then underwent XLIF for the diagnosis of LSS. Disc height was restored and the symptom was released after the procedure (**Fig. 7.8**).

Degenerative scoliosis is also a good indication for XLIF technique. A 49-year-old female patient was diagnosed with deformity in the lower back since 4 years and progressed with intermittent claudication. She underwent a stage surgery. XLIF was performed at three levels as the first stage, and 1 month later, a posterior correction surgery was performed that reduced the curve from initial 56.6 to 6.9 degrees, and symptoms were released (**Fig. 7.9**).

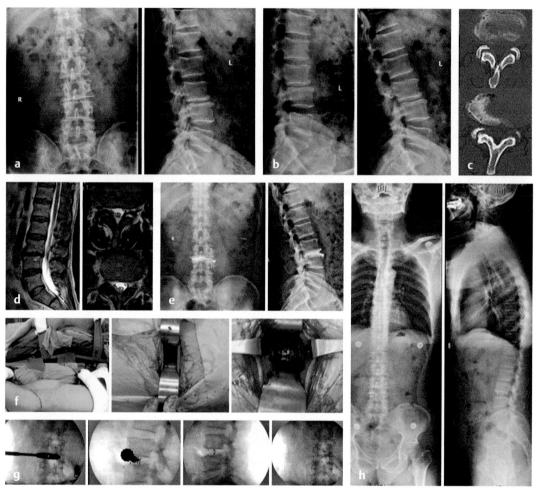

Fig. 7.8 X-ray anteroposterior view of lumbar spine demonstrating reduction of disc height and vertebra slip at L3/4 **(a)**; extension and flexibility of X-ray demonstrating instability at L3/4 **(b)**; CT-scan and MRI showing stenosis at L3/4 **(c, d)**; the responsible level was determined by discography **(e)**; body position, intraspinal images, and cage inserted **(f, g)**; postoperative full-length spine film **(h)**.

Postoperative Care

Patients with the XLIF technique should be encouraged to walk on the same operative day to aid their recovery in muscle function and strength. Postoperative pain tends to be minimal due to the minimally invasive characteristics of the XLIF technique. Therefore, the patients may be discharged after only an overnight hospital stay. Authors recommend that patients should wear lumbar brace for at least 3 months until the fusion is complete.

Clinical Results

Fusion rates are reported well around 90% for the XLIF technique.[6–8] Rodgers et al demonstrated a fusion rate of 93.2% with an average follow-up of 17.3 months via the XLIF technique.[8] Berjano et al described a fusion rate of 98% through the XLIF in a series of 77 patients.[7] Malham et al reported a fusion rate of 85.3% for XLIF at 1-year follow-up.[6]

XLIF is considered as an effective treatment for restoring and/or increasing foraminal height

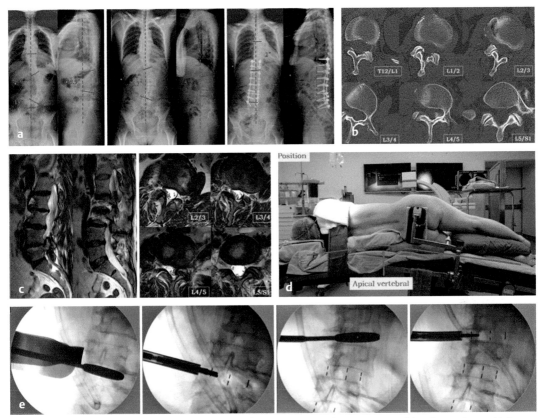

Fig. 7.9 Full-length spine film of preoperative showing a 56.6-degree curve of lumbar spine, which was corrected to 26.7 degrees after staged extreme lateral interbody fusion procedure at L2/3, L3/4, and L4/5, and staged posterior fusion was achieved and the curve was reduced to 6.9 degrees **(a)**. CT scan and MRI demonstrated spinal stenosis at L4/5 of the left side **(b, c)**. Concave approach was determined for first stage correction by extreme lateral interbody fusion **(d, e)**.

to decrease the compression of nerve root. Alimi et al reported a series of 145 XLIF surgeries in which the foraminal height increased by an average of 2.5 mm.[9] Oliveira et al demonstrated an increase of 13.5% foraminal height in their series of 43 XLIF surgical levels.[10] Malham et al described that the foraminal height after 2-day surgery was increased 38% in 79-level XLIF operations.[11] Caputo et al found that the neuroforaminal height was increased up to 80.3% in 30 patients with degenerative lumbar scoliosis via the XLIF technique.[12]

Some researchers believed that XLIF with unilateral or bilateral pedicle screw fixation could increase lumbar lordosis, and bilateral fixation provided greater stabilization.[13–15] Alimi et al reported that XLIF plus unilateral pedicle/screw fixation effectively resolved radicular symptom and maintained increased unilateral

foraminal height after around 11-month operation in patients with unilateral symptomatic vertical foraminal stenosis.[13] Fogel et al compared the efficacy of XLIF standalone cages versus XLIF with various fixation methods in seven cadavers at the L4–5 level, and finally they concluded bilateral pedicle screws could provide the greatest stability.[14] Phillips et al obtained consistent results with Fogel's study in their 107 patients with degenerative scoliosis treated via the XLIF technique plus internal fixations.[15]

The restoration of sagittal balance is beneficial to maintain segmental lordosis. The XLIF technique has a great ability to restore the coronal balance, such as the treatment of degenerative scoliosis. In current studies, some authors believed that the XLIF operation has the ability to improve lumbar lordosis.[16] Watkins et al reported 2.2-degree lordotic correction via

XLIF in their series.[17] Sharma et al and Acosta et al have also demonstrated similar lordotic improvement of 2.8 and 2.9 degrees, respectively.[18,19] However, some authors found that XLIF could only significantly improve lumbar lordosis at L4/5 of 2.4 degrees.[12]

Complications

The most common complications of the XLIF technique are neurological complications, especially transient thigh and groin paresthesias secondary to temporary injury of genitofemoral. It is reported that the incidence rate of paresthesias after XLIF was 0.7 to 62.7%.[20–23] Most patients with paresthesias improve during 4 to 12 weeks after operation, and the paresthesias improves with more than 90% recovery at 1-year postoperatively.[20–23] The rate of transient quadriceps or psoas weakness was reported from 1 to 24% after the XLIF surgery.[8,20,22] The XLIF operated at L4/5 has a high-risk rate of neurological injury due to a variable degree of clearance with respect to traversing nerves. Cummock et al described a higher rate of thigh pain, numbness, and weakness after XLIF at L4–5 level. To decrease the relative higher neurological complications at this level, some surgeons began to take some positive measures. For example, Rodgers et al demonstrated that there was a significant lower rate of paresthesias in patients with intraoperative 10 mg of IV dexamethasone compared with patients who did not undergo the treatment during XLIF of the L4–5 level.[8] In addition, a study showed that there were 13.8% plexus injuries, 0.7 to 33.6% motor deficits, 12.5 to 25% anterior thigh pain, major vascular injuries, bowel perforations and seromas after the XLIF technique.[24]

To decrease or avoid neurological injury after the XLIF technique, it is necessary to perform meticulous dissection, decrease the tension of the muscles, and carry out gentle dilation during the operation course. A cadaveric study showed that a potential injury of the genitofemoral nerve can happen during the transpsoas K-wire and dilator placement. The other nerve roots could be at risk while dissecting via trans psoas approach.[25] Neurological monitoring is an effective way to decrease the incidence of nerve injury and increase safety of the XLIF technique.

Moreover, authors should try best to perform the dilation carefully which should not be larger than the minimum demand for discectomy at targeted level. At last, the proper "breaking" or bending the bed has been theorized to avoid the risk of ipsilateral lumbar plexus injury. Some surgeons believe that the ipsilateral limb pain, weakness, or numbness are more likely to be caused by stretching the lumbar plexus during positioning.

Conclusion

The XLIF technique is an effective treatment for various degenerative lumbar diseases. It has been demonstrated that it is able to acquire a satisfactory result in fusion rates and segmental alignment. Meticulous operation (dissection and dilation) is very important to decrease the incidence of relevant complications, especially at L4–5 level, and surgeons should also pay more attention for specific indications and contradictions of the XLIF technique. Authors believe that the minimally invasive characteristic of the XLIF technique has a bright future pertaining to the treatment of degenerative lumbar diseases, and it is also eligible for The Enhanced Recovery After Surgery Society concepts.

Authors believe that the minimal invasive characteristics of the XLIF technique has a bright future pertaining to the treatment of degenerative lumbar diseases, and it is also eligible for ERAS (Enhanced Recovery After Surgery Society concepts).

References

1. Winder MJ, Gambhir S. Comparison of ALIF vs. XLIF for L4/5 interbody fusion: pros, cons, and literature review. J Spine Surg 2016;2(1):2–8
2. Ozgur BM, Aryan HE, Pimenta L, Taylor WR. Extreme lateral interbody fusion (XLIF): a novel surgical technique for anterior lumbar interbody fusion. Spine J 2006;6(4):435–443
3. Lang G, Perrech M, Navarro-Ramirez R, et al. Potential and limitations of neural decompression in extreme lateral interbody fusion-a systematic review. World Neurosurg 2017;101:99–113
4. Rodgers WB, Lehmen JA, Gerber EJ, Rodgers JA. Grade 2 spondylolisthesis at L4-5 treated by XLIF: safety and midterm results in the "worst case scenario". ScientificWorldJournal 2012;2012: 356712

5. Tessitore E, Molliqaj G, Schaller K, Gautschi OP. Extreme lateral interbody fusion (XLIF): a single-center clinical and radiological follow-up study of 20 patients. J Clin Neurosci 2017;36:76–79

6. Malham GM, Parker RM, Blecher CM, Chow FY, Seex KA. Choice of approach does not affect clinical and radiologic outcomes: a comparative cohort of patients having anterior lumbar inter-body fusion and patients having lateral lumbar interbody fusion at 24 months. Global Spine J 2016;6(5):472–481

7. Berjano P, Langella F, Damilano M, et al. Fusion rate following extreme lateral lumbar interbody fusion. Eur Spine J 2015;24(Suppl 3):369–371

8. Rodgers WB, Gerber EJ, Patterson J. Intraoperative and early postoperative complications in extreme lateral interbody fusion: an analysis of 600 cases. Spine 2011;36(1):26–32

9. Alimi M, Hofstetter CP, Cong GT, et al. Radiological and clinical outcomes following extreme lateral interbody fusion. J Neurosurg Spine 2014;20(6):623–635

10. Oliveira L, Marchi L, Coutinho E, Pimenta L. A radiographic assessment of the ability of the extreme lateral interbody fusion procedure to indirectly decompress the neural elements. Spine 2010;35(26, Suppl):S331–S337

11. Malham GM, Parker RM, Goss B, Blecher CM, Ballok ZE. Indirect foraminal decompression is independent of metabolically active facet arthro-pathy in extreme lateral interbody fusion. Spine 2014;39(22):E1303–E1310

12. Caputo AM, Michael KW, Chapman TM, et al. Extreme lateral interbody fusion for the treat-ment of adult degenerative scoliosis. J Clin Neurosci 2013;20(11):1558–1563

13. Alimi M, Hofstetter CP, Tsiouris AJ, Elowitz E, Härtl R. Extreme lateral interbody fusion for unilateral symptomatic vertical foraminal stenosis. Eur Spine J 2015;24(Suppl 3):346–352

14. Fogel GR, Turner AW, Dooley ZA, Cornwall GB. Biomechanical stability of lateral interbody implants and supplemental fixation in a cadaveric degenerative spondylolisthesis model. Spine 2014;39(19):E1138–E1146

15. Phillips FM, Isaacs RE, Rodgers WB, et al. Adult degenerative scoliosis treated with XLIF: clinical and radiographical results of a prospective multicenter study with 24-month follow-up. Spine 2013;38(21):1853–1861

16. Malham GM, Ellis NJ, Parker RM, et al. Maintenance of segmental lordosis and disk height in stand-alone and instrumented extreme lateral interbody fusion (XLIF). Clin Spine Surg 2017;30(2):E90–E98

17. Watkins RG IV, Hanna R, Chang D, Watkins RG III. Sagittal alignment after lumbar interbody fusion: comparing anterior, lateral, and transforaminal approaches. J Spinal Disord Tech 2014;27(5):253–256

18. Sharma AK, Kepler CK, Girardi FP, Cammisa FP, Huang RC, Sama AA. Lateral lumbar interbody fusion: clinical and radiographic outcomes at 1 year: a preliminary report. J Spinal Disord Tech 2011;24(4):242–250

19. Acosta FL, Liu J, Slimack N, Moller D, Fessler R, Koski T. Changes in coronal and sagittal plane alignment following minimally invasive direct lateral interbody fusion for the treatment of degenerative lumbar disease in adults: a radio-graphic study. J Neurosurg Spine 2011;15(1):92–96

20. Cummock MD, Vanni S, Levi AD, Yu Y, Wang MY. An analysis of postoperative thigh symptoms after minimally invasive transpsoas lumbar interbody fusion. J Neurosurg Spine 2011;15(1):11–18

21. Moller DJ, Slimack NP, Acosta FL Jr, Koski TR, Fessler RG, Liu JC. Minimally invasive lateral lumbar interbody fusion and transpsoas approach-related morbidity. Neurosurg Focus 2011;31(4):E4

22. Khajavi K, Shen A, Hutchison A. Substantial clinical benefit of minimally invasive lateral interbody fusion for degenerative spondylolisthesis. Eur Spine J 2015;24(Suppl 3):314–321

23. Bergey DL, Villavicencio AT, Goldstein T, Regan JJ. Endoscopic lateral transpsoas approach to the lumbar spine. Spine 2004;29(15):1681–1688

24. Epstein NE. Extreme lateral lumbar interbody fusion: do the cons outweigh the pros? Surg Neurol Int 2016;7(Suppl 25):S692–S700

25. Banagan K, Gelb D, Poelstra K, Ludwig S. Anatomic mapping of lumbar nerve roots during a direct lateral transpsoas approach to the spine: a cadaveric study. Spine 2011;36(11):E687–E691

Chapter 8

Anterior Lumbar Interbody Fusion: Indications, Technique, and Complications

8 Anterior Lumbar Interbody Fusion: Indications, Technique, and Complications

Andrew K. Chan, Alvin Y. Chan, Justin M. Lee, Joshua J. Rivera, Vivian P. Le, Praveen V. Mummaneni

Introduction

Anterior lumbar interbody fusion (ALIF) is an anterior approach used for treating a variety of lumbar disease (e.g., spondylolisthesis, degenerative disease, spinal deformity, adjacent segment disease, and flat back syndrome).[1]

There are multiple benefits to an anterior approach. First, ALIF provides robust anterior support for the vertebral column, which provides the majority of axial loading. Second, the anterior approach allows for release of the anterior longitudinal ligament (ALL) and annulus fibrosis. In doing so, the surgeon can use sequential interbody trials as dilators to widen the disc height and correct deformities by indirectly opening the foramen via distraction and restoring the natural lordosis of the lumbar spine.[2] When compared with the posterior approach, ALIF also avoids injury or manipulation of the thecal sac, nerve roots, posterior musculature, and posterior tension band. An anterior approach may also be more likely to prevent adjacent segment disease by avoiding disruption of the posterior muscular tension band.[3] An anterior approach can be used for either single or multiple levels. ALIFs can also be done in isolation or in conjunction with posterior fixation (i.e., 360-degree approach). Here, authors review the indications, technique, and complications associated with anterior lumbar interbody fusion.

Indications and Contraindications

ALIFs should be performed in well-selected patients with lumbar symptoms refractory to conservative medical management. These symptoms can include severe back pain, worsening deformity, progressive instability, or neurological deficits. Indications for ALIF include the need to (1) restore natural disc space height, (2) decompress the neural elements indirectly from loss of disc height, (3) release the ALL or make a wide discectomy to restore lordosis. Relative contraindications include patients with atherosclerotic intra-abdominal vascular calcification (e.g., aortic calcification) and prior retroperitoneal surgery or irradiation. An experienced vascular surgeon may be consulted to assist with the approach.

There may be advantages to ALIF over other types of lumbar interbody fusions. For example, a study of 57 patients undergoing either ALIF or transforaminal lumbar interbody fusion (TLIF) evaluated the difference between the two procedures in terms of restored foraminal height, disc angle, and restored lumbar lordosis.[4] The results were that the ALIF increased foraminal heights by 18.5% compared with 0.4%, and increased disc angle and lordosis while TLIF decreased both parameters. However, there is evidence that ALIF may result in higher rates of readmissions and costs compared with TLIF or posterior lumbar interbody fusions. The surgeon must use proper judgment when determining which procedures to use.[5] The patients who may benefit most are those who require ALL release and correction of lumbar kyphosis.

Preoperative Planning

There are several preoperative images that should be obtained prior to surgery. Anterior–posterior (AP) and lateral radiographs, including flexion and extension views, are typically obtained to identify areas of instability. Additionally, AP and lateral 36-inch scoliosis films may be used to evaluate scoliosis and global sagittal and coronal balance to ensure that the construct placed optimizes segmental and regional balance. Next, a magnetic resonance imaging (MRI) scan should be obtained to evaluate for areas of disc herniation or central canal or foraminal stenosis. In patients with prior abdominal surgeries, it may be useful to obtain abdominal imaging (e.g., abdominal radiograph, computed tomography [CT], or MRI with angiography). Additionally, CT with vessel imaging may be obtained preoperatively to evaluate for abnormal vasculature, severe atherosclerosis, or atypical organ locations.

The spine surgeon should either be experienced and comfortable with the anterior approach as well as its complications, or an approach surgeon may assist to minimize complications. An ALIF done without intraoperative complications typically results in minimal blood loss (<100 mL). However, preparing for catastrophic blood loss in the rare event of vascular injury is important. Preoperatively, type and cross-matched blood is often held for potential transfusion. Multiple points of intravenous access should be obtained in preparation for transfusion. An arterial line may be inserted for hemodynamic monitoring. The appropriate surgical instrumentation for controlling severe hemorrhage from injured vasculature (a rare event) should be available in the operating room and identified prior to the start of the case.

Surgical Steps

Operative Setup

The patient is first placed and secured in the supine position; authors prefer to place a small positioning bump beneath the L5–S1 junction. Additionally, the patient may be placed in slight Trendelenburg if the L5–S1 disc is to be removed. Authors then ensure appropriate padding of the pressure points, avoiding any possible pressure-related injuries. A pulse oximeter is placed on the left big toe, allowing for iliac vessel blood flow assessment during the surgery. A sterilely draped C-arm is placed above the patient to give the surgeon better access. C-arm fluoroscopy is used for localizing the target level to help pinpoint where the incision should be made.

Surgical Technique

An anterior abdominal paramedian incision—on the lateral border of the rectus abdominus—is made vertically on the left (authors' preference), allowing retroperitoneal access. Of note, a right-sided incision may be made allowing for a right retroperitoneal approach in patients who have had prior left abdominal surgery with scar tissue. A longitudinal incision of the lateral border of the anterior rectus sheath is authors' preference but for L5–S1 a Pfannenstiel incision is also acceptable; a muscle paralytic medication (e.g., rocuronium) can be used to help with exposure if necessary to relax the abdomen. The posterior rectus sheath and transversalis fascia are divided below the arcuate line. Below this line, the layers of the abdominal wall must be divided slowly. This includes the anterior layer of the rectus sheath, the rectus abdominis muscle, the transversalis fascia, and the extraperitoneal fascia. Once the incision is dissected down to the peritoneum, blunt dissection is used to access the retroperitoneal space. The vertebral bodies should be exposed along with the left psoas muscle laterally. Important vessels (e.g., common or left iliac artery and veins) should be gently dissected and retracted away from the field. Then, a retractor system is utilized to maintain exposure (**Fig. 8.1**). The retractor may need adjustments if changes in the plethysmograph on the big toe are encountered.

Managing the vessels depends on the disc level. If the levels are more superior (e.g., L2–3, L3–4), the left segmental artery and vein should be divided and the aorta, iliac artery, and vein should be mobilized to the right.

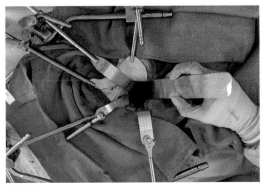

Fig. 8.1 A retractor system used for the anterior lumbar interbody fusion approach.

At L4–5, the iliolumbar vein (left-side segmental vein) should be identified and also divided due to the high risk of avulsion when the left common iliac vein is mobilized. Bleeding can be difficult to control if the vessel is avulsed. The iliac vessels should be retracted to the right. This should be done cautiously because the left external iliac artery is at risk of compression during this maneuver. In addition, the external iliac pulse may be palpated when the retractor is moved.

The L5–S1 level is most unique in terms of encountered vasculature. The median sacral vessels are likely to be encountered midline and should be divided. The retractors should be positioned to create a working corridor between the iliac arteries and veins. Importantly, the disc space should be exposed with blunt dissection to avoid injury to the hypogastric plexus, which may cause retrograde ejaculation.

Before performing the disc dissection, fluoroscopy should be used to ensure appropriate localization of the disc level (**Fig. 8.2**). An annulotomy is then made to penetrate to the disc space. The annulotomy is made with the edges along the inferior and superior vertebral body end plates. A Cobb elevator is used to develop the plane between the disc and end plate. The disc is resected via pituitary rongeurs and curettes, while the end plates are prepared using curettes and rasps. The posterior longitudinal ligament may be resected carefully if the patient requires decompression of the canal or neural elements. The remainder of the intervertebral space should be cleared of cartilage and disc material in preparation of inserting the interbody construct.

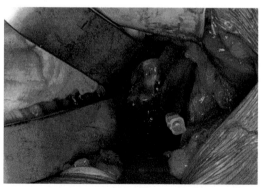

Fig. 8.2 A spinal needle and fluoroscopy are utilized to ensure appropriate localization of the disc level.

Once the intervertebral space is prepared, interbody trials are placed sequentially in terms of size to gradually widen the disc space height until the desired lordosis is created (**Fig. 8.3a–c**). Then, the corresponding interbody implant is prepared with bone graft (e.g., autograft, allograft) and/or bone morphogenetic protein and placed into the intervertebral disc space (**Fig. 8.4**). Implant selection is at the discretion of the surgeon and dictated by the primary goals of surgery (e.g., restoring segmental lordosis and restoration of foraminal height). Authors do prefer the use of titanium implants in the setting of infection. The implant may be affixed to the vertebral bodies using a form of screw fixation to reduce the risk of migration. Of note, if posterior fixation is planned, it is often extended to include the level of the ALIF interbody to increase the fusion rate. Fluoroscopy should be utilized to confirm that the graft is in appropriate position and that the desired lordosis was obtained (**Fig. 8.3d and e**).

After confirming the positioning of the implant, adequate hemostasis must be obtained. The anterior rectus sheath is then closed with a running suture, and the subdermal layers and skin are sutured per surgeon's preference.

Complications

There are several complications that can occur during the procedure for which the surgeon must be prepared.[6] The most common include approach-related ones: vascular injury, lymphocele, retrograde ejaculation via injury to the hypogastric plexus, and injury to the ureter. The most commonly injured vessels include the iliac veins or iliolumbar vein during vessel retraction. Other complications include postoperative ileus, damage to the viscera, an enterocutaneous fistula, abdominal wall protrusion or hernia, as well as retroperitoneal hematomas. The best way to manage these complications is to prevent them by using an access surgeon when the primary surgeon feels unfamiliar with the region. Otherwise, consulting vascular or general surgery or urology may be advisable in managing these complications when they arise. Unrelated to the anterior approach, there is a risk of implant failure, pseudarthrosis, or graft subsidence. The complication rate has been

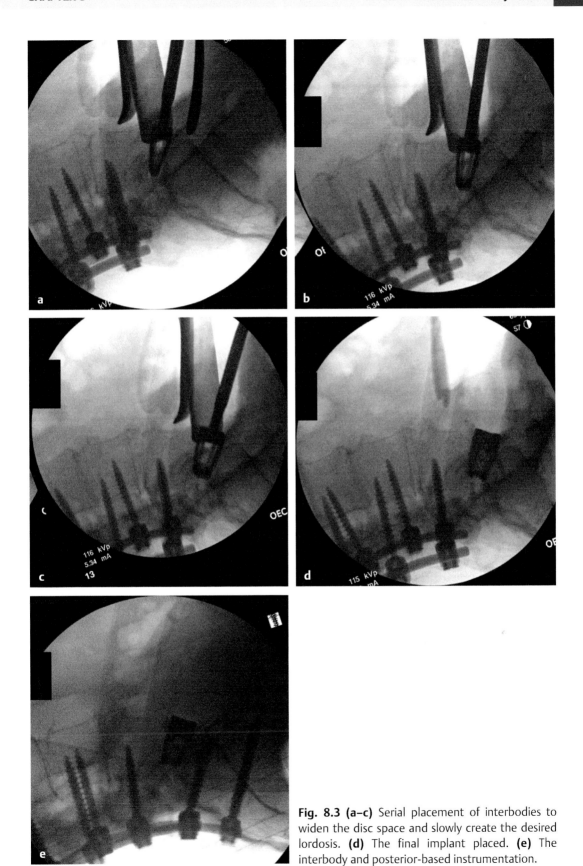

Fig. 8.3 (a–c) Serial placement of interbodies to widen the disc space and slowly create the desired lordosis. **(d)** The final implant placed. **(e)** The interbody and posterior-based instrumentation.

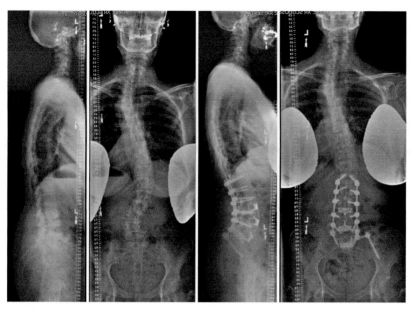

Fig. 8.4 The final interbody implant is inserted into the intervertebral disc space.

estimated to be roughly 10%, though the risk of severe vascular injury is low.[7,8]

In some cases, revision of ALIF is necessary. There is limited literature discussing the operative options, but there is evidence that revision can be safe and effective. A study of 218 open ALIF approaches showed that nine required revisions (~4%), with seven undergoing anterior revision and two requiring a combined approach.[9] There were early complications in four patients, including dural tear, mild neurological deficits, and retrograde ejaculation; the authors argued that although there were no major complications, there may be an increased risk of early complications.

Tips and Tricks

- An approach surgeon may be helpful to deal with a vascular injury complication.

- Prior to the surgery, abdominal imaging should be obtained to evaluate for abnormal anatomy (e.g., unusual vasculature, solitary kidney, etc.).

- Circumferential release of the vertebral bodies may be considered to achieve the desired lordosis. Posterior fusion can be done openly or via minimally invasive techniques depending on the preference and need for osteotomy.

- Most patients will benefit from a left-sided Pfannenstiel or vertical lateral rectus incision and approach for ALIF (to avoid manipulation of the iliac veins which are less sturdy than the iliac arteries). Those who have scar from prior left-sided abdominal surgery may be approached from the right side.

References

1. Chan AK, Mummaneni PV, Shaffrey CI. Approach selection: multiple anterior lumbar interbody fusion to recreate lumbar lordosis versus pedicle subtraction osteotomy: when, why, how? Neurosurg Clin N Am 2018;29(3):341–354

2. Kaiser MG, Haid RW Jr, Subach BR, Miller JS, Smith CD, Rodts GE Jr. Comparison of the mini-open versus laparoscopic approach for anterior lumbar interbody fusion: a retrospective review. Neurosurgery 2002;51(1):97–103, discussion 103–105

3. Min JH, Jang JS, Lee SH. Comparison of anterior- and posterior-approach instrumented lumbar interbody fusion for spondylolisthesis. J Neurosurg Spine 2007;7(1):21–26

4. Hsieh PC, Koski TR, O'Shaughnessy BA, et al. Anterior lumbar interbody fusion in comparison with transforaminal lumbar interbody fusion: implications for the restoration of foraminal height, local disc angle, lumbar lordosis, and sagittal balance. J Neurosurg Spine 2007;7(4):379–386

5. Kureshi SA, Wilkins RH. Posterior fossa reexploration for persistent or recurrent trigeminal

neuralgia or hemifacial spasm: surgical findings and therapeutic implications. Neurosurgery 1998;43(5):1111–1117

6. Sasso RC, Best NM, Mummaneni PV, Reilly TM, Hussain SM. Analysis of operative complications in a series of 471 anterior lumbar interbody fusion procedures. Spine 2005;30(6): 670–674

7. Garg J, Woo K, Hirsch J, Bruffey JD, Dilley RB. Vascular complications of exposure for anterior lumbar interbody fusion. J Vasc Surg 2010; 51(4):946–950, discussion 950

8. Mobbs RJ, Phan K, Daly D, Rao PJ, Lennox A. Approach-related complications of anterior lumbar interbody fusion: results of a combined spine and vascular surgical team. Global Spine J 2016;6(2):147–154

9. Gumbs AA, Hanan S, Yue JJ, Shah RV, Sumpio B. Revision open anterior approaches for spine procedures. Spine J 2007;7(3):280–285

Chapter 9
Oblique Lumbar Interbody Fusion

9 Oblique Lumbar Interbody Fusion

Yu Liang

Introduction

Lumbar interbody fusion is a widely accepted technique for the treatment of degenerative disc disease (DDD). Within a long period of time, posterior lumbar interbody fusion (PLIF) has been playing a predominant role in this field.[1] Associated studies confirmed that PLIF technique is a promising procedure, which showed satisfying outcomes for the lumbar stenosis and disc herniation combined with/or lumbar segmental instability. Transforaminal lumbar interbody fusion (TLIF) technique was introduced to overcome the shortcomings of PLIF, which involves retraction of the nerve root and dura sac. TLIF was first described by Harms and Rolinger in 1982[2] with the benefits of direct decompression of exiting and traversing root and providing three columns support, which is definitely crucial for segmental fusion. However, these posterior approach techniques need relatively wider exposure with inevitability of paraspinal muscles lesion by lifting the muscle attachment from the spinal process, laminar, facet joints, etc.[3]

The spine surgeons started to turn to the lateral lumbar approach. In 1997, Mayer[4] reported 25 patients with lumbar degenerative disease treated by anterior approach to reach a solid fusion with microscope assistance. This has been considered as a prelude of lateral lumbar interbody fusion (LLIF). More recently, Pimenta et al[5] popularized the lateral approach to interbody fusion, or extreme lateral interbody fusion (XLIF). The LLIF is suitable for lumbar spine conditions which require access to the interbody disc space from T12/L1 to L4/5.[6,7] In recent years, several papers associated with LLIF have been published and most of them believe that the technique can be used in the entire spectrum of lumbar degenerative conditions, including DDD with segmental instability, lumbar stenosis, adjacent segment disease, lumbar spondylolisthesis, degenerative scoliosis, lumbar nonunion, etc.

At more caudal levels of the lumbar spine, the lumbar plexus courses more anteriorly and the iliac vessel courses more laterally, which increases the risk of injury via a lateral approach. The patient is positioned laterally, either left or right side depending on surgeon's preference and ease of access. A small lateral incision is performed based on the position and angulation of the disc on image intensification when the patient is positioned. Neuromonitoring is essential for the transpsoas access to the disc space.[7–9]

Oblique lumbar interbody fusion (OLIF) is similar to LLIF, which avoids extended stripping of spinal or paraspinal musculature and direct nerve root decompression.[10,11] This is also called anterior to psoas (ATP) technique, meaning the procedure is accomplished through the ATP corridor.[12,13] With the modification, the lumbar plexus is unlikely to be directly disrupted and complications associated to plexus harassing are reduced. Obviously, L4/5 disc space is therefore much more likely possible to be managed using OLIF than LLIF technique.[14,15] However, potential risks involved with OLIF surgery include sympathetic dysfunction and vascular injury may increase. OLIF25 technique is not suitable for the L5/S1 level, due to the location of the iliac crest that obstructs lateral access. A few papers proposed OLIF51 to deal with the L5/S1 disc space, but the technique and significance remain controversial.[16,17]

Indications

OLIF is likely to cover all the lumbar degenerative condition spectrum. The common indications are as follows.[18–20]

Discogenic Lower Back Pain

OLIF is favorable in disc space preparation and thus with higher fusion rate compared to those of posterior approach surgeries such as PLIF/TLIF.

Lumbar Stenosis

In patients with lumbar foraminal stenosis secondary to narrowed disc space, OLIF is an effective option compared to PLIF/TLIF. This is due to indirect decompression of the foramen with good restoration of disc height.

Degenerative Spondylolisthesis

More recent studies show that with LLIF, lumbar spine alignment can be restored by means of distracting the slipped disc space and indirectly decompressing the nerve structure.

Adjacent Segment Disease

For adjacent segment disease (ASD) after lumbar fusion, OLIF provides a safer solution from anterolateral approach to deal with disc space instead of manipulating through epidural scar, which tremendously reduces the dura tear and nerve root injury.

Degenerative Scoliosis/ Kyphoscoliosis

Considering the much larger size of LLIF cages, the procedure is effective in correcting both coronal and sagittal imbalance by achieving better alignment balance and improved outcomes.

OLIF may also be used for spinal pseudarthrosis/nonunion after posterior spine fusion surgery. During the repeated surgery, the spine surgeons would easily get to the target spine segment to take out the previous fusion cage and to properly manage disc space. Once the disc space preparation is finished, a bigger and stronger fusion cage is then implanted. The trajectory of the OLIF is perpendicular to that of PLIF/TLIF; the disc space height can be maintained effectively and the environment is much

favorable than the posterior repeated surgery (**Figs. 9.1–9.5**).

Contraindications

- Previous retroperitoneal surgery: These include lateral or anterior lumbar spine surgery, kidney surgery, etc.
- Patients with a concave coronal deformity on the right side are not suited for a right prepsoas approach due to the location of the inferior vena cava, which is more likely to develop vascular injury.
- Lack of an operative corridor (on preoperative imaging showing vascular or visceral structures impeding access) is also a contraindication for this procedure. A space must exist between the psoas and the aorta at the level of interest.[15,19]

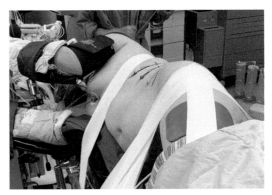

Fig. 9.1 Right lateral decubitus position of a patient for performing oblique lumbar interbody fusion.

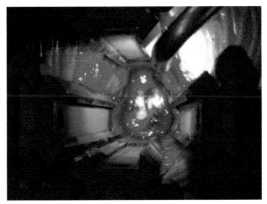

Fig. 9.2 Intraoperative surgical image of the localized level of interest confirmed by imaging.

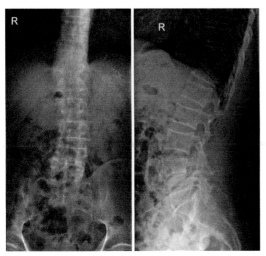

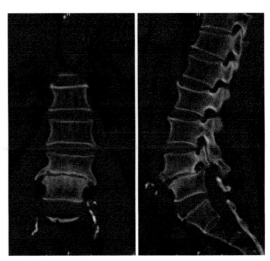

Fig. 9.3 Radiography image of a patient showing completely collapsed disc space at L4–5 level.

Fig. 9.4 Computed tomography scan demonstrating lysis of L4 vertebrae with vacuum sign and collapsed L4–5 disc space.

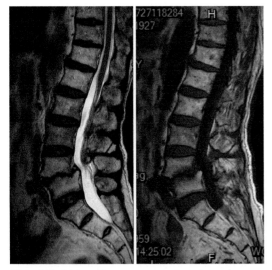

Fig. 9.5 Magnetic resonance imaging demonstrating modic changes in the end plate of L4–5 and spondylolisthesis at the same level with canal stenosis.

Surgical Technique

Preoperative Planning

It is important to collect the patient's information as much as possible, including chief complaint, history of present condition, fundamental diseases, drug allergy history, etc. The surgeon must weigh the risks and benefits the

patient will get from the surgery.[19,21] Making an individualized plan based on image reading (X-ray, MRI, CT scan) is the key point for a successful OLIF surgery. On MRI, the corridor between the vena cava/iliac veins and the disc space needs to be evaluated. If the patient is not able to have an MRI examination, CT scan can be an optional examination. Standing radiographs (EOS is preferable) are to be used to evaluate spinopelvic alignment and the position of the iliac crest, while flexion/extension radiographs are used to evaluate segmental stability and abnormal movement.

Patient Positioning

The patient is induced with general anesthesia and intubated. Long-acting paralytics should not be used as it interferes with application of intraoperative neuromonitoring. The patient is placed in a right side lateral decubitus position with the left side up and the operating table is slightly tilted backward about 20 to 30 degree. An axillary roll is placed along the chest wall, below the axilla, to protect the brachial plexus. All prominent points are meticulously padded and the patient's trunk is held by sticky tape directly to the operation table. The pelvis and chest must be perpendicular to the (horizontal) operating table. A neutral position of the legs relaxes the psoas muscle and allows for easier retraction (**Fig. 9.1**).

Neuromonitoring

In OLIF, the working corridor is anterior to the psoas and some authors no longer consider neuromonitoring as mandatory. Others show a different understanding. Although the risk of femoral nerve injury is low, free run electromyogram and motor evoked potential can alert the surgeon if the lumbar plexus is being compromised. Somatosensory evoked potential can be useful as an additional modality to address false-positive results.

Surgical Approach

Along the iliac crest, a true lateral site is marked and a measurement of 5 cm is marked anterior to this point. This marks the incision for the oblique approach. In case of L4–5 procedure, if the patient has a high iliac crest, the incision may be done 2 cm anterior to the regular incision site.

The incision is made obliquely, parallel to the trajectories of the abdominal wall nerve roots, followed by exposing and splitting the external oblique, internal oblique, and transversus abdominus myofascial layers. Attention should be paid while splitting the transversus abdominis from posterior to anterior so as to reduce the risk of peritoneal perforation. The retroperitoneal fat is seen deep to the transverse abdominis muscle. Finger dissection is used to sweep the retroperitoneal fat and peritoneal contents off the posterior abdominal wall and over the psoas muscle.

The psoas can be gently mobilized posteriorly. The disc space is cleared off soft tissues using blunt instruments. Sequential dilators will be placed and triggered EMG is used to confirm an adequate distance from the lumbar plexus. A table-mounted retractor is then inserted and locked into place. A gentle posterior retraction of the psoas muscle belly is often adequate to allow sufficient exposure of the lumbar segments. Once the surgical levels are identified using fluoroscopy (**Fig. 9.2**), sequential discectomy is performed. Annulotomy using sharp knife is followed by the use of Cobb elevators and curettes to evacuate the disc material under direct visualization and with extreme attention to protect the vertebral end plates.

Thorough discectomy is performed and end plates are prepared. A Cobb elevator is used to break through the contralateral annulus. The interbody cages, of appropriate dimensions, are packed with bone graft material, and placed with low impact. This confirm correct trajectory and placement spanning the apophyseal ring. Fluoroscopy is used to verify interbody position if navigation shifted during the operation. Direct inspection of the retroperitoneal space is performed when the retractor is slowly removed. The wound is then closed in a layered fashion.

L5/S1 Disc Space

The OLIF procedure may be described as a laterally positioned traditional ALIF retroperitoneal approach. However, OLIF51 requires much less dissection of the retroperitoneal space and can be done with a smaller incision using semi-constrained retractors. Associated literatures are reaching consensus that OLIF51 used to get comparable clinical outcomes without taking an additional incision.

Clinical Outcomes

OLIF is a relatively new technique that lacks a large number of clinical studies and a long-term follow-up data. Nevertheless, current cadaveric and clinical studies showed favorable outcomes compared with the other procedures.

Molloy et al[22] reported a clinical study with a relatively short follow-up period and limited number of patients. He concluded that anterolateral technique was noted to be safe with no vascular, neurological, or visceral injuries encountered. The ATP technique, similar to ALIF and lateral LIF, can be used to achieve lumbar fusion in numerous spinal conditions such as recurrent disc herniation, spondylolisthesis, adult spinal deformities, and pseudarthrosis. Potential advantages of the ATP, over ALIF and LLIF, include the ability to approach the entire lumbar spine including the L5–S1 and the thoracolumbar junction through one incision. The prevertebral vessels are hereby identified under direct visualization, and the ALL is safely exposed allowing for anterior column release.

Degenerative Spondylolisthesis

Disc height restoration, foraminal decompression, and correction of lumbar lordosis can be achieved with the ATP technique, similar to LLIF and ALIF. These results are superior to PLIF and with less average blood loss.[23]

Lumbar Stenosis

For lumbar stenosis, especially caused by narrow disc space and secondary foraminal stenosis, indirect decompression of OLIF can play an important role in the treatment, which distracts the disc space and foramen. An appropriate knowledge that OLIF is not suitable for central stenosis or stenosis secondary to bony occupation is necessary.[24,25]

Degenerative Adult Deformity

Great sagittal and coronal deformity correction can be achieved using the anterolateral access when compared to the standard posterior approach. In certain patients, avoiding the need for standard posterior osteotomy is another virtue of the anterior column release that can be achieved by the anterolateral exposure. In a radiographic analysis of 94 patients treated with ATP for multilevel spinal deformities, authors noted an average of additional 25.15 degree of lumbar lordosis correction (over the base line lordosis) and an average of 20.03 degree of coronal Cobb angle correction at 20-months follow-up. Many authors confirmed that the OLIF technique cannot only shorten the fixation segments but can also effectively create spinal lordosis by means of ALL resection and lordotic cage insertion. This can also be named as anterior column realignment (ACR). Staged surgery is favorable for the reason that it gives the surgeon an additional opportunity to re-evaluate the spine alignment after the first stage surgery and to modify the surgical planning accordingly.[18,26,27]

Salvage Surgery

OLIF has been reported to be a better option for repeat surgeries such as pseudarthrosis. Orita mentioned that an anterior approach for salvage surgery is useful; in that it does little harm to intracanal neural tissues by achieving indirect decompression followed by spontaneous recovery of intervertebral and foraminal height. It is suitable for this purpose, as it achieves minimally invasive anterior interbody fusion. Anterior salvaging is also reasonable; in that it avoids additional muscle damage and neurological risks inherent to the posterior approach, with much less blood loss achieved by blunt dissection.[28,29]

Adjacent Segment Disease

ASD is one of the common complications after the spinal fusion surgery. OLIF technique can be used to deal with this condition by standalone or combining with percutaneous pedicle screw system. OLIF technique solves the adjacent segment stenosis and instability with indirect decompression and fusion from lateral approach which avoid dissection through epidural fibrosis, thus reducing the neurological complications, such as dura tear and nerve root injury.[20,30]

Complications

Few associated complications have been reported for OLIF procedure.[31-33] The complications can be divided into different catalogs by the approach-related, cage-related, and other complications. Further, approach-related complications can be divided into neurological, visceral, and other injuries.

Neurological Injuries

1. Motor nerve injury

   Fujibayashi et al[31] reported 1% motor nerve injuries rate compared to 1.1% for XLIF. There was no significant difference between these two techniques.

2. Sensory Nerve Injury

   The authors reported a rate of 3.5% for OLIF while 5.9% for XLIF.[31] This significant difference is due to ATP approach, which avoids injury to the lumbar plexus passing through the psoas instead of a transpsoas approach as in XLIF surgery. Generally, the sensory lesion will disappear 2 to 3 months after the surgery.

3. Sympathetic Trunk Injury

The occurrences of sympathetic trunk injury vary with different clinical researches. Fujibayashi et al[31] reported no occurrence for OLIF procedure while 0.1% for XLIF. Jin et al[34] reported in total 4 patients with sympathetic chain symptom out of 63 patients.

Visceral Injury

1. Ureteral Injury

This is a relatively rare complication with occurrences of 0.3[31] and 0.6%[35] depending on different studies. In 2017, it seems that Lee et al[36] reported the first ureteral injury in OLIF surgery. The author concluded that additional care while manipulating the retroperitoneal fat layer during the OLIF approach can prevent injury to the ureter. The surgeon should suspect ureteral injury, if there are any of the common presenting symptoms and signs, including abdominal pain, flank pain, fever, nausea, vomiting, urinary leakage from the vagina, hematuria, and leukocytosis. Kubota et al[37] published a case report of insidious intraoperative ureteral injury as a complication of OLIF in the same year. The author mentioned that ureter injury is a rare but possible complication of OLIF. Careful use of surgical instruments is the key for preventing intraoperative complications, including ureteral injury. Delayed contrast-enhanced CT and retrograde urography are useful form of the diagnosis of the injury.

2. Bowel injury

This is a rare but fatal complication of OLIF. Fujibayashi et al reported zero occurrence while 0.05% for the XLIF and other LLIF techniques.[31] If the bowel is violated, it should be repaired urgently.

Vascular Injury

This mainly consists of major vascular injury, segmental artery injury, and retroperitoneal hematoma. In a report of 2,998 cases from Japan,[31] the major vascular injury was 0.03% for OLIF. For segmental artery injury, it was 0.3% with XLIF and 0.7% with OLIF. This difference was not significant. In a comparative study of DLIF and OLIF, there was no significant difference for the local hematoma with 4.5% for DLIF and 4.8% for OLIF. The others showed no difference as well with various lateral techniques (0.3% for OLIF and 0.1% for XLIF).

Others

The other visceral injuries include pleural laceration, diaphragm laceration, lung injury, etc., which are of low incidence but severe and sometimes fatal. Surgeons should be aware of those possibilities and should be ready to handle.

1. Cage Related

A. Cage Subsidence (Vertebral Body Fracture)

Cage subsidence or vertebral body fracture is not rare (2.2–18.7% for OLIF). This complication which is caused by the preparation of the end plate or placement of the cage, requires additional procedure such as posterior percutaneous pedicle screw fixation to avoid segmental stability.

B. Cage Malpositioning

Cage malpositioning occurs in 0.3% of surgeries. This includes front-to-back misalignment, migration to opposite side, and anterior dislodgement. The patient has to be revised when there is neurological impairment or instability.[31]

Conclusion

OLIF is a true minimally invasive technique with many advantages compared to the other lumbar fusion procedures such as avoidance of the paraspinal muscles injury, strong support to the anterior column, larger fusion surface, reliable correction, and reduction ability, etc. It is getting more popular among the spine surgeons in recent times. However, attention must be paid to the negative aspect as well. One should be aware of the complications of OLIF, which are possible and sometimes fatal. Strict training program and cadaver study can reduce complication occurrence.

Tips and Tricks

- A proper patient selection for OLIF in lumbar spine disease is the most important predictor of good postoperative outcomes.

- An adequate (>10 mm) oblique window between aorta and psoas muscle is essential for a safe procedure.

- Orthogonal maneuver should be performed only after reaching at least half the distance of the vertebral body in the mediolateral plane for appropriate positioning of the cage.

References

1. Briggs H, Milligan PR. Chip fusion of the low back following exploration of the spinal canal. J Bone Joint Surg Am 1944;26:125–130

2. Harms J, Rolinger H. A one-stager procedure in operative treatment of spondylolistheses: dorsal traction-reposition and anterior fusion (author's transl) [article in German]. Z Orthop Ihre Grenzgeb 1982;120(3):343–347

3. Mobbs RJ, Sivabalan P, Li J. Minimally invasive surgery compared to open spinal fusion for the treatment of degenerative lumbar spine pathologies. J Clin Neurosci 2012;19(6):829–835

4. Mayer HM. A new microsurgical technique for minimally invasive anterior lumbar interbody fusion. Spine 1997;22(6):691–699, discussion 700

5. Pimenta L, Vigna F, Bellera F, Schaffa T, Malcolm J, McAfee P. A new minimally invasive surgical technique for adult lumbar degenerative scoliosis. Paper presented at: Proceedings of the 11th International Meeting on Advanced Spine Techniques (IMAST); July 2004; Southampton, Bermuda

6. Ozgur BM, Aryan HE, Pimenta L, Taylor WR. Extreme lateral interbody fusion (XLIF): a novel surgical technique for anterior lumbar interbody fusion. Spine J 2006;6(4):435–443

7. Malham GM, Ellis NJ, Parker RM, Seex KA. Clinical outcome and fusion rates after the first 30 extreme lateral interbody fusions. ScientificWorldJournal 2012;2012:246989

8. O'Brien JR. Nerve injury in lateral lumbar interbody fusion. Spine 2017;42(Suppl 7):S24

9. Cummock MD, Vanni S, Levi AD, Yu Y, Wang MY. An analysis of postoperative thigh symptoms after minimally invasive transpsoas lumbar interbody fusion. J Neurosurg Spine 2011;15(1):11–18

10. Fujibayashi S, Hynes RA, Otsuki B, Kimura H, Takemoto M, Matsuda S. Effect of indirect neural decompression through oblique lateral interbody fusion for degenerative lumbar disease. Spine 2015;40(3):E175–E182

11. Davis TT, Hynes RA, Fung DA, et al. Retroperitoneal oblique corridor to the L2-S1 intervertebral discs in the lateral position: an anatomic study. J Neurosurg Spine 2014;21(5):785–793

12. Tannoury C, Tannoury T. Anterolateral retroperitoneal psoas sparing (anterior to psoas: ATP) lumbar interbody fusion for degenerative spine and adult deformity: surgical technique and the evidence. Semin Spine Surg 2018;4:237–246

13. Silvestre C, Mac-Thiong JM, Hilmi R, Roussouly P. Complications and morbidities of mini-open anterior retroperitoneal lumbar interbody fusion: oblique lumbar interbody fusion in 179 patients. Asian Spine J 2012;6(2):89–97

14. Sato J, Ohtori S, Orita S, et al. Radiographic evaluation of indirect decompression of mini-open anterior retroperitoneal lumbar interbody fusion: oblique lateral interbody fusion for degenerated lumbar spondylolisthesis. Eur Spine J 2017;26(3):671–678

15. Mobbs RJ, Phan K, Malham G, Seex K, Rao PJ. Lumbar interbody fusion: techniques, indications and comparison of interbody fusion options including PLIF, TLIF, MI-TLIF, OLIF/ATP, LLIF and ALIF. J Spine Surg 2015;1(1):2–18

16. Chung NS, Jeon CH, Lee HD. Use of an alternative surgical corridor in oblique lateral interbody fusion at the L5-S1 segment: a technical report. Clin Spine Surg 2018;31(7):293–296

17. Kim JS, Sharma SB. How I do it? Oblique lumbar interbody fusion at L5S1(OLIF51). Acta Neurochir (Wien) 2019;161(6):1079–1083

18. Anand N, Kong C, Fessler RG. A staged protocol for circumferential minimally invasive surgical correction of adult spinal deformity. Neurosurgery 2017;81(5):733–739

19. Orita S, Inage K, Furuya T, et al. Oblique lateral interbody fusion (OLIF): indications and techniques. Oper Tech Orthop 2017;27:223–230

20. Jin C, Xie M, He L, et al. Oblique lumbar interbody fusion for adjacent segment disease after posterior lumbar fusion: a case-controlled study. J Orthop Surg Res 2019;14(1):216

21. Mehren C, Korge A. Minimally invasive anterior oblique lumbar interbody fusion (OLIF). Eur Spine J 2016;25(Suppl 4):471–472

22. Molloy S, Butler JS, Benton A, Malhotra K, Selvadurai S, Agu O. A new extensile anterolateral retroperitoneal approach for lumbar interbody

fusion from L1 to S1: a prospective series with clinical outcomes. Spine J 2016;16(6):786–791

23. McGowan JE, Kanter AS. Lateral approaches for the surgical treatment of lumbar spondylolisthesis. Neurosurg Clin N Am 2019;30(3):313–322

24. Beng TB, Kotani Y, Sia U, Gonchar I. Effect of indirect neural decompression with oblique lateral interbody fusion was influenced by preoperative lumbar lordosis in adult spinal deformity surgery. Asian Spine J 2019 (e-pub ahead of print). doi:0.31616/asj.2018.0283

25. Mehren C, Mayer HM, Zandanell C, Siepe CJ, Korge A. The oblique anterolateral approach to the lumbar spine provides access to the lumbar spine with few early complications. Clin Orthop Relat Res 2016;474(9):2020–2027

26. Anand N, Cohen RB, Cohen J, Kahndehroo B, Kahwaty S, Baron E. The influence of lordotic cages on creating sagittal balance in the CMIS treatment of adult spinal deformity. Int J Spine Surg 2017;11:23

27. Buell TJ, Chen CJ, Nguyen JH, et al. Surgical correction of severe adult lumbar scoliosis (major curves ≥ 75°): retrospective analysis with minimum 2-year follow-up. J Neurosurg Spine 2019;21:1–14

28. Phan K, Mobbs RJ. Oblique lumbar interbody fusion for revision of non-union following prior posterior surgery: a case report. Orthop Surg 2015;7(4):364–367

29. Orita S, Nakajima T, Konno K, et al. Salvage strategy for failed spinal fusion surgery using lumbar lateral interbody fusion technique: a technical note. Spine Surg Relat Res 2018;2:86–92

30. Sakamoto T, Abe K, Orita S, et al. Three cases of adjacent segment disease post-posterior spinal fusion, treated successfully by oblique lateral interbody fusion: a clinical series. Clin Case Rep 2018;7(1):206–210

31. Fujibayashi S, Kawakami N, Asazuma T, et al. Complications associated with lateral interbody fusion: nationwide survey of 2998 cases during the first 2 years of its use in Japan. Spine 2017;42(19):1478–1484

32. Tannoury T, Kempegowda H, Haddadi K, Tannoury C. Complications associated with minimally invasive anterior to the psoas (ATP) fusion of the lumbosacral spine. Spine 2019 (e-pub ahead of print). doi:10.1097/BRS.0000000000003071

33. Walker CT, Farber SH, Cole TS, et al. Complications for minimally invasive lateral interbody arthrodesis: a systematic review and meta-analysis comparing prepsoas and transpsoas approaches. J Neurosurg Spine 2019;25:1–15

34. Jin C, Jaiswal MS, Jeun SS, Ryu KS, Hur JW, Kim JS. Outcomes of oblique lateral interbody fusion for degenerative lumbar disease in patients under or over 65 years of age. J Orthop Surg Res 2018; 13(1):38

35. Abe K, Orita S, Mannoji C, et al. Perioperative Complications in 155 Patients Who Underwent Oblique Lateral Interbody Fusion Surgery: Perspectives and Indications From a Retrospective, Multicenter Survey. Spine 2017;42(1):55–62

36. Lee HJ, Kim JS, Ryu KS, Park CK. Ureter Injury as a Complication of Oblique Lumbar Interbody Fusion. World Neurosurg 2017;102:693.e7–693. e14

37. Kubota G, Orita S, Umimura T, Takahashi K, Ohtori S. Insidious intraoperative ureteral injury as a complication in oblique lumbar interbody fusion surgery: a case report. BMC Res Notes 2017;10(1):193

Chapter 10
Implants and Biologics in Lumbar Interbody Fusion

10 Implants and Biologics in Lumbar Interbody Fusion

Komal Prasad Chandrachari

Introduction

Lumbar interbody fusion (LIF) is an established surgical technique for various degenerative conditions affecting the lumbar spine. It is also indicated in other pathologies such as trauma, infection, and neoplasia. LIF procedure involves placement of an implant (cage, spacer, or graft) within the intervertebral space after discectomy and end plate preparation.[1] The fusion is generally performed using one of the five main open approaches: posterior LIF (PLIF), transforaminal LIF (TLIF), oblique LIF (OLIF), anterior LIF (ALIF), and lateral LIF (LLIF) or by using minimally invasive (MIS) or endoscopic approaches. There is no explicit evidence available to show that one of these methods is superior over others. Also, there is no clear-cut evidence to suggest whether bony fusion rates positively correlate with better clinical outcomes.[2] The evolution of interbody fusion techniques parallels the advances in implants and biologics designed to restore near-normal anatomy. In this chapter, the author intends to discuss the evolution of cages, the different materials used for interbody fusion ranging from auto- to allografts, and biological implants.

Principles of Bone Fusion

Bone is a dynamic tissue that is constantly renewed and remodeled. Following injury, bone heals by a process where active cells and minerals form a rigid framework for load bearing. Physical activity, biomechanics, hormones, nutritional status, and other medical comorbidities influence the process of bone fusion. The physiological processes influencing the incorporation of bone graft[3] are compiled in **Table 10.1**.

Osseointegration is the stable anchorage of an implant achieved by direct bone-to-implant contact. Osseointegration is also histologically defined in Dorland's Illustrated Medical Dictionary as the direct anchorage of an implant by the formation of bony tissue around the implant without the growth of fibrous tissue at the bone–implant interface.[4] Bone tissue adapts to the load it bears. Wolff's law suggests that some amount of loading is helpful to induce bone remodeling to achieve arthrodesis.

Autograft bone has all the properties for successful bony fusion—osteogenesis, osteoinduction, and osteoconduction. It contains viable osteoblasts and osteoprogenitor cells for osteogenesis. Endogenous bone morphogenetic proteins (BMPs) are osteoinductive. Osteoconduction is facilitated by similar bone quality of the autograft at the recipient site. In addition, they have no antigenic potential. Therefore, autografts remain the gold standard for LIF. Anterior iliac crest, posterior iliac crest, fibula, and rib are the most common sources for autograft. Local autograft from laminar decompression can be also used, but it has a high proportion of cortical bone. There will be an initial

Table 10.1 Physiological properties of bone grafts

Physiology	Description	Materials
Osteogenesis	New bone formation through cellular proliferation	Fresh autologous bone graft containing bone-forming osteoprogenitor cells
Osteoinduction	Stimulation of precursor cells to differentiate into mature bone	Demineralized bone matrix (DBM) and bone morphogenetic protein (BMP) are potent osteoinductors
Osteoconduction	Growth of bone on a surface or a three-dimensional scaffold	Materials with pores such as Ceramics; need autograft for solid bone fusion

phase of bone resorption followed by a phase of creeping substitution. Complete remodeling and bony fusion takes about a year. The advantages of using autografts include a high fusion rate, availability, no implant cost, and no disease transmission.[5] However, autografts can have certain disadvantages such as donor site pain, wound dehiscence, infection, hematoma, fracture of the ileum, sensory disturbance, and cosmetic impairment.

LIF techniques have several proven advantages over onlay grafting because of a decreased incidence of pseudoarthrosis, accelerated rate of fusion, and increased axial load-bearing ability. Interbody implants when placed optimally along the neutral axis reduce significant bending. These implants may be composed of bone, non-bone materials, or a combination of both, such as interbody cages. The use of autografts alone, as demonstrated by Cloward, had produced poor results with high mortality and morbidity.[5] This led to the development and predominant use of cages in regular practice.

The Evolution of Cages

Bagby designed the first cage implant for cervical myelopathy in racehorses. Kuslich et al adapted the "Bagby basket" for human use in late 1980s. It included use of a threaded hollow titanium cylinder with thick perforated wall and cancellous bone chips placed in the hollow. Bagby and Kuslich (BAK) cage was first implanted in humans in 1992 using a posterior approach. It was later adapted for anterior approaches also that were used in LIF.[6] Ray modified the BAK cage with deeper threads to promote "self-tapping." Cylindrical mesh cage, with rolled titanium mesh filled with autograft and reinforced with rings at both ends, was introduced in 1986 by Harms and Biederman. In due course of time, the cylindrical cages were replaced by wider implants to increase the axial strength and reduce subsidence. It was followed by wedge-shaped, lumbar-tapered cages which were developed to allow restoration of sagittal alignment.

The Ideal Lumbar Intervertebral Cage

Normal lordotic curve of the lumbar spine is predominantly contributed by L4 to S1 segments. The trapezoidal shape of L5 vertebra contributes to lordosis. About an additional 12 degree of lordosis is due to the shape of the L4–L5 disc. Further ~15 degree is added by L5–S1 disc. The purpose of lumbar intervertebral cages is to reconstruct the sagittal alignment of lumbar spine. It is notable that most of the indications for performing an LIF have associated loss of lordosis also.

An ideal lumbar interbody cage recreates adequate disc space, restores intervertebral lordosis and foraminal height. It also provides substantial area for fusion to take place and restore normal anatomy. The height of LIF cage will restore the disc height and widen the neural foramina. Lumbar lordosis can be restored by choosing appropriate height and wedging of LIF cage. Width and breadth of the implant is important to widen the area available for bony fusion. Smaller implant will limit the area of bony fusion and reduce stability. Larger implant may damage the adjacent structures.

Classification of Lumbar Interbody Fusion Devices

Lumbar interbody implants can be broadly classified as either replacement devices or fusion devices. While lumbar interbody replacement devices aim to maintain motion at the disc segment, fusion devices aim to obliterate any such motion. Further interbody fusion device classification is shown in **Table 10.2**.

Based on Approach

TLIF and PLIF procedures involve discectomy, end plate preparation, and the cage insertion in a narrow corridor requiring retraction of the dura. This leads to higher risk of dural tear and nerve injury. Support of tactile feedback and

Table 10.2 Classification of interbody fusion devices

Classification	Types
Based on purpose	Fusion devices Replacement devices
Approach of insertion	Anterior Oblique Lateral Posterior Axial
Type of material	PEEK Titanium alloy Hybrid
Dynamicity	Static Dynamic
Degree of lordosis	Neutral Lordosis Hyperlordosis

Abbreviation: PEEK, polyether ether ketone.

fluoroscopy are necessary for placement of the cage through these approaches. This limitation of space means that the interbody cages used with posterior approaches are smaller compared with those used for ALIF/OLIF/LLIF. Being small, they do not span from end to end of the vertebral body and usually rest in the central portion of lumbar end plate, susceptible to subsidence. Further, with MIS approaches, the visualization is more challenging.

To allow traversing the narrow corridor of insertion, the cage is devised to be of trapezoid or "bullet" shaped. Bilateral approach is required in PLIF for symmetric placement of another bullet cage. To avoid opening the annulus on opposite side, bullet cage is asymmetrically placed unilaterally too. "Boomerang"- or "banana"-shaped cages are fashioned to place the cage more centrally using a unilateral approach in TLIF. Cage size, shape, and position, in addition to surgical technique, determine lordosis during PLIF/TLIF surgery. Anterior placement with enough "clear space" behind the cages is recommended by Landham et al.[7] In a study of 83 patients undergoing single-level PLIF, they noted that placement of the paired cages should be relatively anterior within the disc space to optimize the lordosis gain. They inferred that when the sagittal midpoint of the

cages is anterior to the midpoint of the disc, the increase in lordosis at the level of reconstruction is optimized.

Takahashi et al studied the importance of cage geometry in determining post-PLIF lumbar lordosis. They found that optimal intervertebral body angle and subsequent lordosis cannot be achieved by cage geometry alone.[8]

Based on Type of Material

Following Bagby cages, surgeons invented different types of cages for various surgeries and most of them were predominantly made of stainless steel. Titanium metal was introduced in 1989, and cages were made of titanium instead of stainless steel. Till now it has stood the test of time, and pedicle screws and cages made of titanium are still in practice. The limitations of titanium cages include its interference with radiological assessment. Stiff titanium cage will also tend to subside into adjacent vertebra.

Polyether ether ketone (PEEK) cages were introduced in 1990s to avoid the disadvantages of titanium cages. It is radiolucent material allowing better radiological assessment of bony fusion. Its elasticity is like that of cortical bone. This promotes even stress distribution leading to lower subsidence rates and possible higher fusion rates (**Fig. 10.1**).

Integral fixation cages have an additional screw system along with cage and plate for stabilizing the motion segment. Integral fixation devices use screws (two, three, or four) to secure implant to the end plates above and below the device to assist implant fixation. This will obviate the need for additional posterior fixation after ALIF.

Heida et al[9] reviewed 29 published reports studying the effect of clinical outcomes of grafts and spacers in TLIF. They assessed fusion rates for three different interbody spacers (CAPSTONE, PEEK Spinal System, and TELAMON) and four different combinations of bone grafts and extenders (locally harvested bone, iliac crest bone with local bone, local bone with recombinant human BMP2 [rhBMP2], and a mixture of local and allograft bone). This study

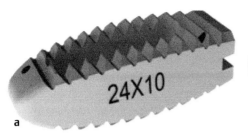
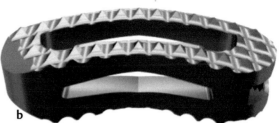

Fig. 10.1 Lumbar interbody fusion devices. **(a)** Bull Cage PEEK (GESCO Healthcare)—posterior lumbar interbody fusion device: bullet nose and smooth edges ensure easy insertion and the anatomical contours and serrated profile ensure good placement between vertebrae and reduces chance of pull-out. **(b)** Bean Cage (GESCO Healthcare)—transforaminal lumbar interbody fusion device: bean-like form ensures a maximized contact area between vertebrae and the implant.

found that CAPSTONE and locally harvested bone alone are relatively superior in terms of fusion rates.

Based on Dynamicity

Though static interbody fusion devices are commonly used, newer technological advances in design have led to emergence of expandable interbody devices. They are narrow in collapsed state during initial insertion, avoiding excessive dural and nerve root retraction. Once inside the disc space, they can be sequentially expanded both vertically as well as horizontally to have a wider footprint.

StaXx XD Expandable Device (Spine Wave, USA), CALIBER (Globus Medica, USA), AccuLIF TL (CoAlign Innovations), SmArtCage-L (SmartSpine SAS) are some examples of newer expandable lumbar interbody devices for posterior approaches. Though early clinical results with the expandable devices are promising, there is limited data to support widespread use. Recently, one of the commercially available devices, Stryker AccuLIF posterior lumbar (PL) expandable cage was removed from the market due to a high rate of subsidence. Hence, further studies are necessary to establish safety of these devices.[10]

Biologic Implants

Threaded bone dowels from freeze-dried femurs or tibias are used as an alternative to titanium cage construct. Bone dowels have unique advantage of transmission of more

physiological forces than titanium. Femoral ring allografts are biological cages made from allograft and machined into wedge-shaped rings. Hollow centers of such ring allografts can be filled with allograft or BMP. Allograft bone is derived from a deceased donor, and the graft is either decontaminated or may undergo a process of sterilization. The methods of processing influence the rate at which a graft will incorporate in the recipient. Allografts may stimulate localized immune response in the recipient and can cause delayed fusion. Freeze-dried preparations decrease graft antigenicity but are more susceptible to longitudinal cracks.

Demineralized bone matrix (DBM) is produced by pulverization and acidic extraction of allograft bone. It contains collagen and growth factors with osteoinductive and osteoconductive properties. However, DBM has no structural strength and is not useful without autograft. Current literature recommends use of DBM as bone graft extenders in conjunction with autograft.

Bone marrow aspirate can be obtained at the time of iliac crest autograft harvesting. The aspirated bone marrow contains pluripotent connective tissue progenitor cells that differentiate into mature osteoblasts resulting in improved bone healing. Several factors, such as blood loss, corticosteroid therapy or alcohol abuse, smoking, and age, can influence the number of osteoprogenitor cells and osteoinduction.[11] The bone marrow aspirate can be mixed with other bone graft extenders such as ceramics for fusion.

Platelet-rich plasma (PRP) is an autologous product with a high concentration of platelets in a small volume of plasma. It has osteoinductive effects and is usually combined with hydroxyapatite (HA) which has osteoconductive ability. PRP contains several kinds of autologous growth factors such as transforming growth factor b1 and platelet-derived growth factor. In rat models, combination of PRP and HA was adequate to complete bone union in LIF and also decrease the inflammatory neuropeptides dorsal nerve root ganglions. A latest study has reported increased fusion rate in human subjects.[12]

Ceramics

Ceramics, such as HA and tricalcium phosphate, have good osteoconductive property. They are brittle and lack structural strength, osteogenicity, and osteoinductivity. Therefore, they are used in conjunction with autografts as graft expanders.[13]

Bone Morphogenetic Proteins

The effective component of extracellular matrix from the degradation of dead bone that has capacity to induce new bone formation was isolated in 1971 and was called BMP. The term BMP now refers to a group of growth factors that have the capability to induce bone or cartilage formation. Originally, 7 such proteins, called BMP-1 through BMP-7, were discovered; 13 other BMPs have also been identified recently. With the advent of recombinant DNA technology, rhBMPs are available for clinical use. Recombinant BMP-7 and rhBMP-2 are most studied and potent among the family of BMPs.

BMPs require a carrier such as collagen sponge or HA for slow, controlled release. Several studies have demonstrated the superiority of rhBMP over autografts and allografts in achieving bony fusion. Bony resorption of implanted grafts, ectopic ossification, and seroma formation are important complications of BMP usage.

In a review of use of BMP in spinal surgeries, Burke et al[14] opined that BMP provides excellent enhancement of fusion in many spinal surgeries. However, they quote that "BMP should be a cautionary tale about the use of industry-sponsored research, perceived conflicts of interest, and holding the field of spinal surgery to the highest academic scrutiny and ethical standards." They felt that lack of a transparent base of literature has led to the unfortunate delays in allowing the superior technology of BMPs to help patients. Hofstetter et al[15] conducted an exploratory meta-analysis of use of BMP in various spinal procedures. They found that the use of BMP enhanced rate of fusion in ALIF. However, there is a higher rate of complications, including retrograde ejaculation. In TLIFs, use of BMP had minimal effect on fusion rates. The rate of adverse events, especially radiculopathy was higher in this group. For PLIF, BMP was shown to enhance fusion with minimal side effects. A systematic review and meta-analysis of 13 randomized control trials and 31 cohort studies on rhBMP2 in spine fusion[16] concluded that rhBMP has no proven clinical advantage over bone graft and may be associated with important side effects such as retrograde ejaculation and urogenital problems.

Newer Materials: Composites, Bioabsorbable Polymers, 3-D Printing, and Nanotexturing

Although PEEK has good mechanical properties, it is chemically inert—a property which limits its ability to osseointegrate into surrounding bone. Integrating PEEK with HA (HA-PEEK) or titanium (Ti-PEEK) creates a composite material that mimics natural bone. Studies have shown better osteointegration with HA-PEEK and Ti-PEEK composite cages. Silicon nitride, tantalum, nitinol (alloy of nickel and titanium) are other materials with potential benefits as LIF cages.[17]

Poly (D, L-lactide-co-glycolide) is a promising polymer experimentally used to produce a bioabsorbable implant that is rigid at implantation but gradually degrades and gets absorbed over time without leaving any foreign material in the disc space. Three-dimensional printed porous titanium alloy was found to have good bony ingrowth potential in sheep model.[18]

Extensive research has shown that osseointegration can be enhanced by changing roughness or coating titanium with a ceramic such as HA. The cellular effects of surface topography in the nanoscale range is described recently.[19] PEEK plus (Vallum Corp) is a new Food and Drug Administration-approved interbody fusion device with 20 to 50 nm concavities on the surface of PEEK cage with improved osseointegration.

Gene therapy may have clinical applications in future by genetic transduction of local host cells for sustained production of bioactive proteins to facilitate bony fusion. Transplantation of mesenchymal stem cells for enhancement of bony fusion is being studied in animal models and in clinical studies.

Limitations of LIF Implants and Biologics

The popularity of LIF implants and biologics is spectacularly disproportionate to the evidence regarding its benefits. Theoretically, a solid bony fusion aided by a suitable interbody device, which has good osseointegrative property, should lead to better clinical outcomes. However, the availability of such ideal material and device for clinical use is elusive. Moreover, studies have failed to correlate better clinical outcomes with solid bony fusion. The complications of LIF implants, such as graft migration and neurological, vascular, and urological injury, should be weighed against its potential benefits.

The cost of LIF implants is another important limitation for its widespread use. Cost-effectiveness studies and value-driven outcome studies in the developed world are also pointing toward guarded usage of LIF implants and biologics.

Conclusion

Major advances have been made over the past decade in implants and biologics in the field of LIF. Current efforts are focused on improving osseointegration and integrated screw cages. Multiple promising new designs are currently being evaluated. However, the inadequate clinical evidence and lack of comparisons between different models have eluded definitive conclusions regarding the advantages and disadvantages of one implant over another. Further studies to identify the ideal osseointegrative and cost-effective LIF implant are required to improve clinical outcomes.

References

1. Mobbs RJ, Phan K, Malham G, Seex K, Rao PJ. Lumbar interbody fusion: techniques, indications and comparison of interbody fusion options including PLIF, TLIF, MI-TLIF, OLIF/ATP, LLIF and ALIF. J Spine Surg 2015;1(1):2–18
2. Hagenmaier HS, Delawi D, Verschoor N, Oner F, van Susante JL. No correlation between slip reduction in low-grade spondylolisthesis or change in neuroforaminal morphology and clinical outcome. BMC Musculoskelet Disord 2013; 14(1): 245
3. Albrektsson T, Johansson C. Osteoinduction, osteoconduction and osseointegration. Eur Spine J 2001;10(2, Suppl 2)S96–S101
4. Dorland WA. Newman 1864–1956. Dorland's Illustrated Medical Dictionary. 32nd ed. Philadelphia, PA: Saunders/Elsevier, 2012
5. Phan K, Mobbs RJ. Evolution of design of interbody cages for anterior lumbar interbody fusion. Orthop Surg 2016;8(3):270–277
6. Mummaneni PV, Meyer SA, Wu JC. Biological approaches to spinal instrumentation and fusion in spinal deformity surgery. Clin Neurosurg 2011; 58:110–116
7. Landham PR, Don AS, Robertson PA. Do position and size matter? An analysis of cage and placement variables for optimum lordosis in PLIF reconstruction. Eur Spine J 2017;26(11):2843–2850
8. Takahashi H, Suguro T, Yokoyama Y, Iida Y, Terashima F, Wada A. Effect of cage geometry on sagittal alignment after posterior lumbar interbody fusion for degenerative disc disease. J Orthop Surg (Hong Kong) 2010;18(2):139–142
9. Heida K Jr, Ebraheim M, Siddiqui S, Liu J. Effects on clinical outcomes of grafts and spacers used in transforaminal lumbar interbody fusion: a critical review. Orthop Surg 2013;5(1):13–17
10. Gussous YM, Jain N, Khan SN. Posterior based lumbar interbody fusion devices: static and expandable technology. Semin Spine Surg 2018; 30(4):203–206
11. Roholl PJ, Blauw E, Zurcher C, Dormans JA, Theuns HM. Evidence for a diminished maturation of preosteoblasts into osteoblasts during aging in rats: an ultrastructural analysis. J Bone Miner Res 1994;9(3):355–366

12. Kubota G, Kamoda H, Orita S, et al. Efficacy of platelet-rich plasma for bone fusion in transforaminal lumbar interbody fusion. Asian Spine J 2018;12(1):112–118

13. Chang KY, Hsu WK. Spinal biologics in minimally invasive lumbar surgery. Minim Invasive Surg 2018;2018:5230350

14. Burke JF, Dhall SS. Bone morphogenic protein use in spinal surgery. Neurosurg Clin N Am 2017; 28(3):331–334

15. Hofstetter CP, Hofer AS, Levi AD. Exploratory meta-analysis on dose-related efficacy and morbidity of bone morphogenetic protein in spinal arthrodesis surgery. J Neurosurg Spine 2016; 24(3):457–475

16. Fu R, Selph S, McDonagh M, et al. Effectiveness and harms of recombinant human bone morphogenetic protein-2 in spine fusion: a systematic review and meta-analysis. Ann Intern Med 2013; 158(12):890–902

17. Rao PJ, Pelletier MH, Walsh WR, Mobbs RJ. Spine interbody implants: material selection and modification, functionalization and bioactivation of surfaces to improve osseointegration. Orthop Surg 2014;6(2):81–89

18. McGilvray KC, Easley J, Seim HB, et al. Bony ingrowth potential of 3D-printed porous titanium alloy: a direct comparison of interbody cage materials in an in vivo ovine lumbar fusion model. Spine J 2018;18(7):1250–1260

19. Chaput CD. Surface treatments for spinal implants: a biological perspective. Spine 2018; 43(7S):S6

Chapter 11
Complications and Revision in Lumbar Interbody Fusion

11 Complications and Revision in Lumbar Interbody Fusion

Kshitij Chaudhary, Arjun Dhawale

Introduction

Interbody fusion can be achieved via posterior lumbar interbody fusion (PLIF) or transforaminal lumbar interbody fusion (TLIF), lateral lumbar interbody fusion (LLIF) or oblique lumbar interbody fusion (OLIF), or anterior lumbar interbody fusion (ALIF) approaches. The advent of newer technologies and refinement of the existing approaches in lumbar interbody fusion, resulted in good postoperative outcomes with minimal blood loss and short hospital stay. However, complications associated with any procedure need attention and awareness among surgeons, so as to prevent them as far as possible. In this chapter, authors will be enumerating complications specific to the technique of interbody fusion. Authors have divided the chapter into two main sections: approach and cage-related complications with a focus on the latter. They will discuss revision strategies related to these complications. And finally, they will briefly mention how to deal with infections of the interbody implant.

Approach-Related Complications

Avoiding approach-related complications is dependent on the surgeon's familiarity with the approach and clear understanding of the anatomical structures which can be encountered with each approach.

Anterior Approach (ALIF)

Due to the anatomical proximity of the great vessels, especially to the L4–5 and L5–S1 discs, vascular injury is probably the most concerning complication of the anterior approach. The incidence of vascular complications varies widely from 0 to 15.6%.[1]

A recent meta-analysis reported the overall complication rate of anterior surgery as 14.1% with intraoperative complication and postoperative complication rates of 9.1 and 5.2%, respectively.[2] There were 3.2% venous injuries, 2.73% retrograde ejaculation, 2% neurological injury, 1% superficial infection, 1.4% postoperative ileus, and 1.3% other complications. Venous injuries are more commonly reported due to retraction of the left common iliac, inferior vena cava, and iliolumbar veins (**Fig. 11.1**). Due to the risk of retrograde ejaculation, the anterior approach should be used selectively in males. Neurological complications include neurological deficits, dysesthesias, and sympathetic dysfunction.[2]

Complication rates have been reported to be higher in laparoscopic and transperitoneal approaches versus mini-open or open anterior retroperitoneal approach. The transperitoneal is associated with a higher rate of retrograde ejaculation and postoperative ileus. An incisional hernia could be a late complication.

The literature is variable on whether an access surgeon reduces approach-related complication rates.[2] However, familiarity with the approach is definitely necessary to minimize complications.

Lateral Lumbar Transpsoas Approach (LLIF)

Lumbar plexus injury is the predominant concern with the lateral transpsoas approach for interbody fusion. The incidence of neurological complications in a recent systematic review is 36.1%, transient hip flexor weakness is 14.1%, transient thigh numbness is 17.1%, and transient thigh pain is 26.5%.[3] There are two specific mechanisms of lumbar plexus injury. The retractor or an instrument can directly injure a nerve in the path of the dissection. Also, a less

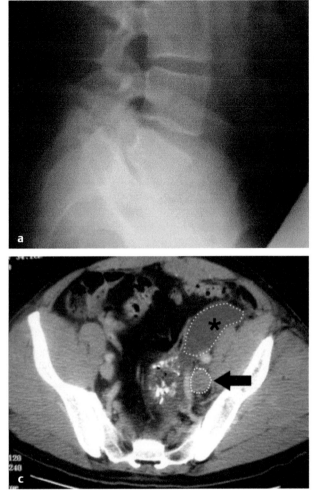

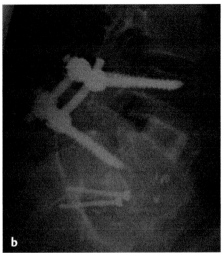

Fig. 11.1 (a) A 38-year-old male with adult isthmic spondylolisthesis underwent. (b) L4–5 and L5–S1 anterior lumbar interbody fusion followed by posterior spinal fusion. (c) He developed retroperitoneal hematoma (*) and venous thrombus (black arrow) from external iliac vein down to proximal calf.

recognized mechanism is an indirect injury caused by prolonged compression of the plexus within the psoas between the posterior retractor blade and the transverse process. Many underplay this problem and claim that most neurological deficits are transient, but the reported rate of permanent neurological damage is as high as 4%, of which quadriceps palsy is the most devastating.[3,4] The risk is higher at L4–5 level as the plexus is more ventrally situated. Prolonged retraction time can also lead to injury. Apart from the knowledge of local anatomy (covered in the chapter), use of neuromonitoring is recommended to avoid neural injury. Free running and triggered EMG is the popular technique that is used. However, this is only a neural proximity monitoring technique and can help with the first mechanism of injury. Indirect injury to lumbar plexus due to prolonged retraction may

not be detected on eletromyographic (EMG) monitoring.[4] Therefore it is recommended that the surgeons should use neural integrity monitoring techniques, like somatosensory evoked potential and motor evoked potential, in addition to EMG.[4]

Vascular injuries may occur but are less frequently reported as compared with the anterior approach. The rate of common iliac vein injury is 0.25%. The use of the temporary pin in the midbody for retraction can result in segmental vessel injury and should be avoided, and the stabilizing pin should be positioned just below the superior end plate. The use of the monopolar cautery should be minimized and bipolar cautery is preferable.[1] Retrograde ejaculation does not seem to a problem with this approach; however, visceral injuries such as bowel, ureter, and renal have been reported sporadically but many such events are under-reported. Pneumothorax and diaphragm injuries can occur while accessing upper lumbar levels.

Oblique Lumbar Interbody Fusion

The OLIF approach theoretically aims to address the approach-related complications of both ALIF and LLIF. By using an oblique surgical corridor between the aorta and anterior border of psoas, OLIF may be able to avoid lumbar plexus injury that is so commonly encountered in the lower lumbar transpsoas approach obviating the need for neuromonitoring the lumbar plexus.[5] However, in addition to visceral injuries as seen with LLIF, OLIF surgery can cause sympathetic dysfunction and vascular injury (0.9%).[5] The most common postoperative complaint, as with LLIF, remains transient weakness, pain, or numbness in the thigh/groin.[6] The risk of retrograde ejaculation seems to be lesser than ALIF. Robust studies directly comparing OLIF and other lateral approaches are unavailable at present. Since it is a relatively new approach, the evidence that OLIF is safer than other lateral approaches is lacking.[6]

PLIF/TLIF

Important approach-related complications of these posterior approaches are dural tears, infections, and nerve damage. A recent meta-analysis comparing the outcomes and complication rates of PLIF and TLIF reported on 990 patients (450 TLIF and 540 PLIF), with an 8.7% complication rate with TLIF versus 17% with PLIF. All complications were higher in the PLIF group. Nerve root damage was reported in 5 patients in the TLIF group and 26 patients in the PLIF group. Dural tears were also more common in the PLIF group, 33 versus 15 in the TLIF group. Infections were higher in the PLIF group with 15 cases versus 7 in the TLIF group.[7]

Cage-Related Complications

Cage Malposition

Cage malposition, as opposed to cage migration (CM), is usually due to an error in the surgical technique. Malposition of the interbody device

out of the confines of the disc could lead to life-threatening complications due to the proximity of important vascular and visceral structures anterolateral to the disc space. Fortunately, it is a rare complication with a reported incidence of 0.26% in PLIF surgeries.[8]

PLIF/TLIF

Ariyoshi et al reported a 74-year-old woman in whom an L4–5 TLIF cage was misplaced too anteriorly that it entered the retroperitoneal space.[9] The cage did not cause a vascular injury then, but when the surgeons tried to retrieve the cage after a week via a retroperitoneal approach, an IVC injury occurred that could not be repaired necessitating a complete ligature of the IVC. Fortunately, the patient survived but had a close brush with death as she bled ~20 L. Pawar et al reported a 55-year-old patient with infective spondylodiscitis in whom the TLIF cage got pushed anteriorly while trying to achieve an optimum position.[10] There was torrential bleeding through the disc space, and the vascular surgeons repaired the IVC injury via an anterior approach but could not find the cage. Later, it was found to have embolized to the left pulmonary artery, surprisingly, without any adverse effect.

Careful attention to technique can avoid this complication. One should never release the cage from the introducer until a lateral fluoroscopic image confirms its location. Once the cage is released, further impaction to achieve "ideal position" using an instrument, like a punch, that is not firmly locked on to the cage, is risky.[11] In addition to lateral fluoroscopy, check the cage position in AP view as well to confirm that it is not too lateral in scoliotic spines as the anatomy can be disorienting. A greater stability will be achieved when the TLIF cage is placed near the vertebral body midline, so that it provides optimal stability in lateral bending in a coronal plane. In the sagittal plane, when the cage is placed anterior and further away from the posterior construct, it provides better stability during flexion and extension.[12-14] Avoid the use of an oversized cage, or impacting the cage without sufficient distraction of the disc space as these situations require very strong impaction that can be uncontrolled. In addition, over distracting the disc space can rupture the anterior longitudinal ligament and annulus, especially in infective spondylodiscitis, allowing the cage to migrate anteriorly if one is not careful.[10] When two PLIF cages are used, the surgeon should be careful while inserting the second cage and make sure that it is not pushing out the first cage anteriorly.

Salvage strategy

If the cage is misplaced anteriorly and the surgeon encounters catastrophic bleeding, assume injury to the great vessels and call for vascular surgeon's help. Sometimes temporary control can be achieved by packing the disc space. If bleeding cannot be controlled, the surgeon must immediately turn the patient supine and control the bleeding via an anterior approach. If no significant bleeding has occurred then one can attempt to retrieve the cage if it is partially within the disc space. Some have successfully achieved this with the help of an arthroscope.[8] If the cage is too anterior, then the surgeon may proceed with the surgery and complete it as long as the hemodynamics are under control. A postoperative computed tomography (CT) angiogram should be sought as early as possible. If the cage is compressing viscera or is touching the great vessels, it should be removed with the help of a vascular surgeon to avoid pseudoaneurysm or organ injury. However, such a call should be taken in consultation with the vascular surgeon, as an anterior approach to retrieve the cage can lead to life-threatening vascular injury and sometimes it may be wiser to leave the cage alone.[11]

LLIF/OLIF

LLIF/OLIF use a narrow surgical corridor and this can limit the visualization of the disc space. Surgeons rely on perfect orthogonal fluoroscopy, meticulous patient positioning, and neuromonitoring to guide cage placement. In cases of anterior procedures like OLIF, the ideal position of a cage is at anterior one-third of the vertebral body to recreate segmental lordosis without compromising on the indirect neural decompression.[15] Here again, a technical error is usually responsible for malpositioned cages. In spite of correct positioning and fluoroscopy, if one fails to appreciate the oval nature of the vertebral body, the surgeon may go out of the

confines of the disc space in the far anterior or far lateral region in the vicinity of the vessels or nerve roots.[16] If the cage is placed obliquely across the disc, the far end could infringe on the contralateral foramen.[17]

Regev et al reported that cage overhang (cage beyond the borders of the disc) could occur if the cage length is determined solely on the basis of AP fluoroscopic image. If the cage is placed in the anterior one-thirds of the disc space, then 45% of the cages are found to have a significant overhang that could potentially compromise the contralateral neural foramen. They recommend using a 15% shorter cage if the cage is placed anteriorly. However, for a more precise fit, the cage length should be measured preoperatively on axial magnetic resonance imaging (MRI) or CT.[16]

The risk of LLIF/OLIF cage malposition is higher in degenerative scoliosis due to axially rotated vertebrae. If the cage is out of the confines of the disc, risk of injury to important structures could be higher as the nerves are more anterior on the convexity and the vessels more in the concavity of the deformity.[16]

Anterior Lumbar Interbody Fusion

ALIF cage malposition is usually because the surgeon fails to identify the midline accurately. This can lead to a laterally positioned cage. If sized incorrectly, then this can compromise the neural foramen. The anterior edge of the cage and blocking screws should be well within the anterior border of the cage to prevent injury to the great vessels.[1]

Cage Subsidence and Migration

Cage migration (CM)—as opposed to malposition—can be defined as a cage that was initially positioned correctly but later moved from its implanted location in the horizontal plane. In an extreme situation, the cage can migrate into the spinal canal or the foramen resulting in cage retropulsion (CR). This horizontal plane movement of the cage can be accompanied by cage subsidence into the end plates.

Migrated lumbar cages with or without subsidence can result in focal kyphosis and mal-alignment (**Fig. 11.2**). Sometimes this can

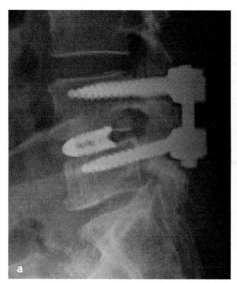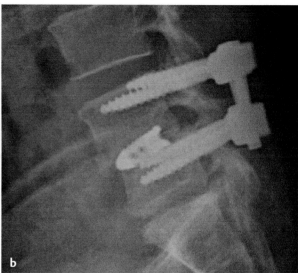

Fig. 11.2 Subsidence of cage with suspected loosening screws 6 months after surgery **(a, b)** but patient is asymptomatic.

prevent successful fusion, which in turn can lead to screw loosening and can aggravate the CM.[18] Not only can the patient experience back pain, but also they can develop neurological symptoms.

PLIF/TLIF Cage Migration

Studies have shown that CM and CR tend to occur relatively in the early postoperative period, usually in the first 3 months of surgery.[19] The risk factors for CM in PLIF/TLIF can be broadly classified as patient-related, radiological, or surgical technique-related factors.[19]

Patient-related factors

1. **Osteoporosis:** Patients with osteoporosis are at a higher risk of cage subsidence and migration.[18] The stability of the cage not only depends on the end plate strength but also on the fixation strength of the pedicle screws (**Fig. 11.3**). Osteoporosis can lead to loosening of the pedicle screws which in turn can result in CM. Although, in many situations, it may be impossible to determine whether the CM/subsidence led to screw failure or vice-versa.

2. **Body mass index:** Whether body mass index (BMI) influences the risk of construct failure is unclear. One would

imagine an obese individual with high BMI to have a higher risk of CM. However, one study found low BMI to be associated with CR, but they could not convincingly explain the mechanism of how high BMI protects the cage.[20]

Radiological factors

The radiological shape of the disc has been found to influence the risk of CM. Some evidence suggests that higher posterior disc height increased the risk of CM.[21] Some have stated that greater preoperative ROM and taller discs have a higher risk of CR.[22] Usually, end plates have a flat or a concave surface such that a cage tends to have maximum contact with uniform load distribution. However, pear-shaped disc has convex-shaped end plates in the posterior half and has a concave shape in the anterior half.[21,22] Such a disc shape does not make contact with all the four corners of the cage in the sagittal plane, which may lead to instability and CM. Therefore, the surgeon should carefully evaluate the shape of the disc space when considering PLIF or TLIF.[21,22]

Surgical technique

1. **Cage-related factors**: *Design*: There are three common types of cage designs—bullet, box, and banana. Bullet-shaped cages, although easy to insert, have been

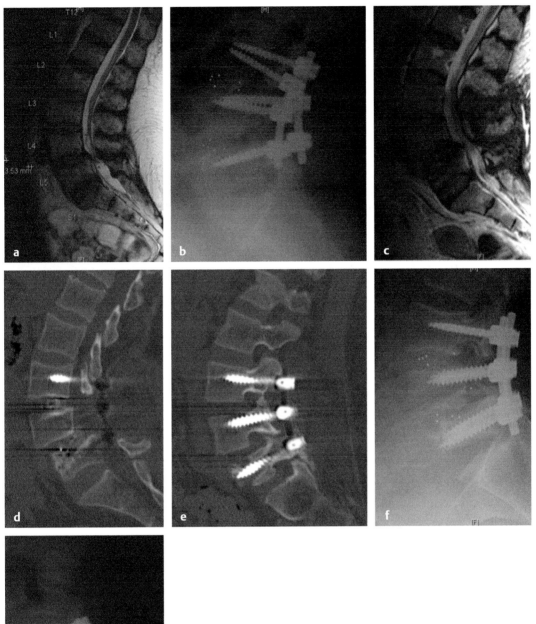

Fig. 11.3 (a) Grade I L4–5 degenerative spondylolisthesis in a 55-year-old man. **(b)** L3–4 and L4–5 transforaminal lumbar interbody fusion (TLIF) was done. Intraoperative surgeon noted that the bone was soft. **(c–e)** After a month, there was acute increase in pain and the patient was unable to mobilize. Magnetic resonance imaging and computed tomography showed L5 superior end plate fracture with loosening of L5 screws. **(f)** The TLIF cage at L4–5 had migrated posteriorly. Anterior approach was not feasible due to previous kidney transplant. Posterior surgery was done. Larger diameter screws were placed in L3 and L4. L5 screws were removed. S1 and iliac screws were used for distal fixation. Bone morphogenetic protein was used for posterolateral fusion. As there was no leg pain, cage removal was not attempted. **(g)** Ten months later, the patients' symptoms resolved and had a successful fusion.

shown to be a risk factor for CR in several studies.[21] The literature is not clear whether the *material* (titanium or PEEK) influences CM. *Size:* Undersized cage for obvious reason can move within the disc space. Over-sized cages will result in end plate injury in addition to the loss of regional lordosis. *Location:* Posteriorly placed cage, identified if the midpoint of the cage is posterior to the midpoint of the disc space, is at a higher risk for retropulsion.[18]

2. **Posterior instrumentation:** Due to high risk of CM, standalone cages are not recommended. However, whether unilateral fixation is sufficient to achieve fusion and prevent CM is controversial but several studies have warned against the use of unilateral fixation due to the high risk of failure.[21] If the posterior instrumentation is not gently compressed over the cage, then there is a risk of CR. This can especially happen in minimally invasive (MIS) TLIF procedures if one is not careful.[23]

3. **Fusion level:** L5–S1 level seems to be especially prone to CR.[22] This level has the most lordosis in the lumbar spine and common cage designs do not have adequate lordosis to achieve an adequate fit.[22] Many times L5–S1 TLIF will be done to protect the S1 screw in a long lumbar fusion. This can put a lot of stress on the S1 screw making this region prone to cantilever failure. The surgeon can choose a banana-shaped cage in a highly lordotic disc and compress on the screws to prevent CM. In addition, iliac fixation can be used to protect the L5–S1 construct in multilevel fusions.

4. **End plate injury:** If end plates are aggressively curetted, especially in osteoporotic bone, then the cage can subside and migrate. End plate should not be violated at the same time the cartilage should be adequately removed.[22] The disc space should be distracted using lamina spreader before hammering the cage in, otherwise trying to force a cage in a collapsed disc space will injure the end plate, predisposing the cage to subside or migrate.

Revision strategy in PLIF/TLIF cage retropulsion

Most patients with CR will require surgery.[19] Posterior revision surgery is technically demanding due to extensive fibrosis and risk of injury to the neural elements while extracting the cage (**Fig. 11.4**). Excessive nerve root retraction can leave the patient with a permanently dysesthetic leg with a palsy. Some have suggested that revision of CR following TLIF might be easier and safer as the cage tends to migrate laterally away from the dural edge.[21] Others have successfully employed a transdural approach to remove the cage instead of retracting the neural elements.[24] Anterior approach to retrieve an interbody cage is also problematic. High incidence of vascular injury has been reported in anterior approaches, especially at L4–5 level, due to perivascular adhesions even when the cage has been inserted via a PLIF/TLIF approach.[25]

LLIF/OLIF Cage Migration

Subsidence is a frequent problem with LLIF with reported incidence from 10 to 60% depending on how one defines subsidence.[3] Although frequently asymptomatic, it can lead to loss of alignment and failure of indirect decompression in addition to pseudarthrosis and possibly revision surgery. Studies have found subsidence to be more common with longer constructs and taller cages. If the cages do not have rim fit, then the cage can sink in, especially if the bone is osteoporotic.

Fortunately, movement of LLIF cage in the horizontal plane (CM) is less frequent, especially as most LLIFs are supplemented with posterior fixation[26] (**Fig. 11.5**). If the contralateral annulus is not adequately released, especially in degenerative scoliosis, residual coronal imbalance may force the cage out from the side it is inserted.[26] The caudal end plate is weaker than the upper end plate, and hence care should be taken not to injure it especially with the Cobb elevator. Protective slides should be used to initiate entry of the cage. Less tall and wider cages are less prone for subsidence or migration.

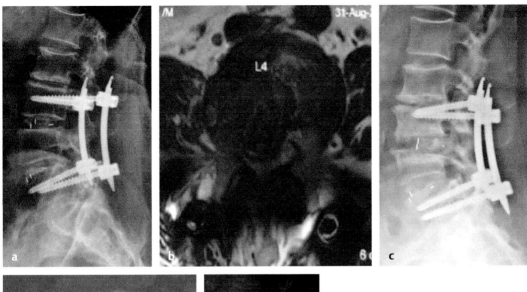

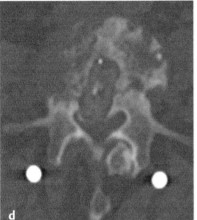

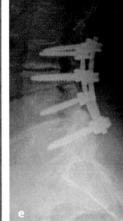

Fig. 11.4 An 82-year-old woman with L3–4 and L4–5 MIS transforaminal lumbar interbody fusion (a). Two years later became symptomatic with severe radiculopathy due to L3–4 nonunion, cage retropulsion, and L3 pedicle screws loosening. Magnetic resonance imaging (c) and computed tomography (d) show cage retropulsion. (e) Posterior revision had to be done with L3–4 cage removal, new cage insertion with bone morphogenetic protein, and extension of fusion to L2.

ALIF Cage Migration

CM after ALIF is a rare event reported in less than 1% of the patients.[2] Sometimes cage dislodgement can occur when the patient is flipped in the prone position for supplemental posterior fixation. The cause is usually a lack of tight fit by an undersized cage/graft that does not adequately tension the annulus. On the contrary, oversizing the cage can also thrust the cage out with or without catastrophic failure of the end plates. As discussed before, osteoporosis can also contribute to the weakened bone–cage interface.

This complication can be avoided by correctly sizing the graft and avoiding damage to the end plates. In spite of improvement in cage design from cylindrical to a box shape, standalone ALIF cages are biomechanically weak

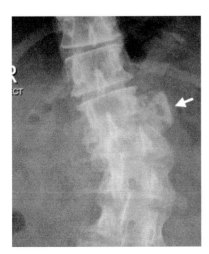

Fig. 11.5 Graft dislodgement in a 65-year-old patient with anterior interbody fusion with iliac crest autograft for pyogenic discitis; no supplementary posterior fixation was done.

and are fraught with cage-related complications. A blocking screw can be placed and some cage designs have interlocking screws that can prevent CM. Anterior plating is another option but they require larger exposure and can have a prominent profile underneath the great vessels. Due to these problems, most surgeons prefer supplemental posterior fixation to avoid these problems.[1]

Pseudoarthrosis

Several studies have reported a high rate of interbody fusion using cages, well over 98%.[3,7] Many interbody nonunions may not be symptomatic; hence, the rate of revision surgery remains acceptably low. Any of the above-mentioned cage complications can lead to a pseudarthrosis; however, fusion may still occur in spite of cage malposition, subsidence, or migration as successful fusion is usually a race between bone healing and implant failure (**Fig. 11.4**). Patient's biology plays an equally important part; general health, nutrition, medications, and smoking-related factors should be evaluated thoroughly.

Infected Interbody Implant

The diagnosis of infection around the interbody cage can be detected on MRI as adjacent bone marrow edema, fluid collection, end plate erosions, and contrast enhancement of remaining disc. Sometimes this can be confused with aseptic loosening of the cage. However, this condition will demonstrate end plate sclerosis, no fluid collection, minimal marrow edema, if any, and no enhancement of remnant disc space. Most early surgical site infection (SSI; <3 months) can be managed with aggressive debridement, which leads to successful salvage of the implants. However, delayed treatment (>3 months) leads to progressive destruction, loosened implants, and reduces the likelihood of implant salvage (**Fig. 11.6**).

Most surgeons agree that pedicle screw instrumentation can be salvaged and retained when treating SSI in posterolateral instrumented fusion. However, there are conflicting recommendations on how to deal with the infection of an interbody implant. Some support

retaining interbody graft or cage, while others propose that retaining the cage can result in failure to control the infection.[27] Biofilm formation on cages has been proposed as one of the mechanisms for failure to eradicate the infection. Bacterial adherence to tantalum is the least, titanium is intermediate, but worst materials for biofilm formation are PEEK and stainless steel.[27]

A recent study reported only 47% successful infection control in patients who had the interbody device retained and most failures were when there was a delay in the diagnosis of infection by more than a month.[27] The study proposed that in patients with interbody space infection, if there are signs of cage or pedicle screw loosening, posterior debridement only could result in high failure rate (**Fig. 11.6**). For such patients, they recommend radical debridement, removal of the cage, and spinal reconstruction. If there are no radiographic signs of loosening and the infection is detected early (<1 month), posterior debridement only will have a good chance of infection clearance. However, if there has been a delay in diagnosis (>1 month), then the success of posterior debridement only is low, and radical debridement with cage removal is necessary (**Figs. 11.7 and 11.8**)

Key Points

- ALIF approach has a signification approach-related complication profile, with vascular injuries being the most troublesome.

- LLIF approach: Lumbar plexus injury has dampened the enthusiasm for this approach.

- OLIF approach is relatively new, and evidence demonstrating its superiority over ALIF or LLIF in terms of approach-related complications is lacking.

- TLIF approach is more prevalent than PLIF approach due to the lesser risk to neural elements and a better complication profile.

- Cage malposition is usually related to poor surgical technique.

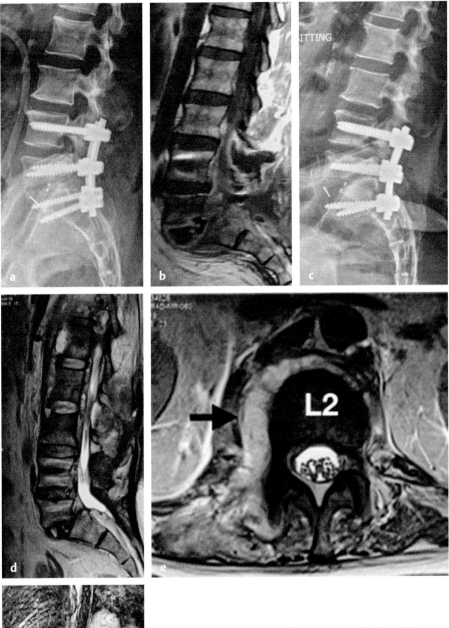

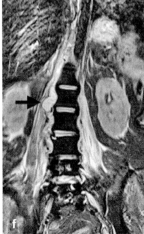

Fig. 11.6 A 55-year-old, diabetic woman developed serious wound infection 1 week after L5–S1 transforaminal lumbar interbody fusion **(a)**. Following debridement, magnetic resonance imaging within a month revealed extensive infection around the cage as well as vertebral bodies **(b)**. The wound healed and the patient was on intravenous antibiotics for 4 months. One year later the S1 screws loosed, L5–S1 spondylolisthesis progressed, and the cage migrated anteriorly **(c)**. Magnetic resonance imaging then showed L5–S1 region with marrow reconstitution but extensive psoas abscess extending superiorly (black arrow) **(d–f)**. This case demonstrates the persistence of infection if the cage is not removed in a patient with loose implants.

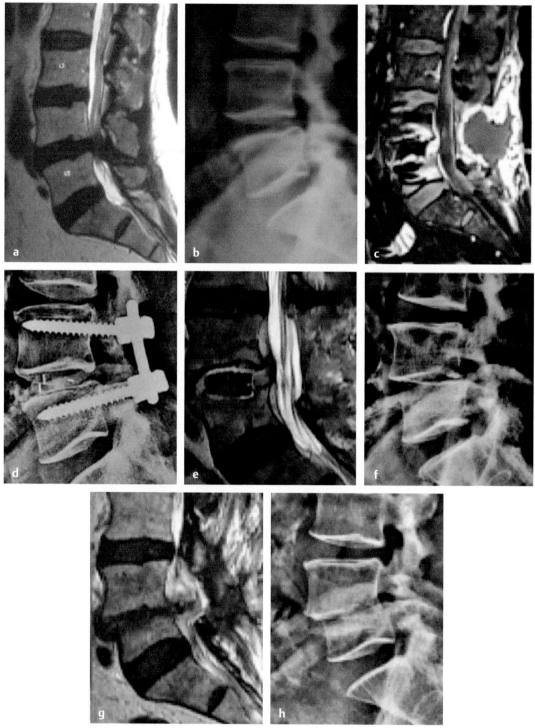

Fig. 11.7 An 80-year-old man underwent L4–5 transforaminal lumbar interbody fusion. Preoperative magnetic resonance imaging (MRI) **(a)** and X-rays **(b)**. He developed deep surgical site infection **(c)**. After repeated debridement and partial implant removal, the infection was still not under control **(d)**. MRI shows persistent infection around the cage **(e)**. Finally the cage was removed **(f)** and then the infection subsided with collapse of the disc **(g, h)**. These images are provided courtesy of Dr. Gautam Zaveri.

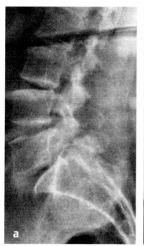
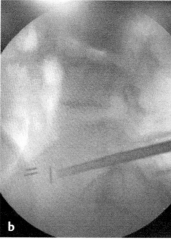
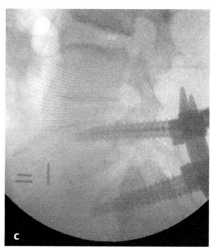

Fig. 11.8 A 70-year-old female with L5-S1 adult isthmic L5/S1 spondylolisthesis was operated for MIS TLIF. **(a)** A 12-mm expandable cage was used. After deployment bone was being packed in the expanded cage. This caused the cage to migrate anteriorly in the retroperiteoneal region **(b, c)**. There was no bleeding. As it was unsafe to retrieve the cage posteriorly, surgeon decided to continue with the surgery. A 12-mm regular cage was placed this time after placing the screws. With the help of an access surgeon the migrated cage was retrieved through a retroperitoneal approach anteriorly. (Image courtesy Dr. Ayush Sharma).

- Cage subsidence is a common occurrence and is not always symptomatic.

- Cage migration can be due to various patient, radiographic, and surgical technique-related factors.

- Infected interbody implants may require aggressive interbody debridement and cage removal if there is an evidence of implant or cage loosening or if the diagnosis of infection is delayed.

References

1. Pichelmann MA, Dekutoski MB. Complications related to anterior and lateral lumbar surgery. Semin Spine Surg 2011;23:91–100

2. Bateman DK, Millhouse PW, Shahi N, et al. Anterior lumbar spine surgery: a systematic review and meta-analysis of associated complications. Spine J 2015;15(5):1118–1132

3. Hijji FY, Narain AS, Bohl DD, et al. Lateral lumbar interbody fusion: a systematic review of complication rates. Spine J 2017;17(10):1412–1419

4. Chaudhary K, Speights K, McGuire K, White AP. Trans-cranial motor evoked potential detection of femoral nerve injury in trans-psoas lateral lumbar interbody fusion. J Clin Monit Comput 2015;29(5):549–554

5. Mobbs RJ, Phan K, Malham G, Seex K, Rao PJ. Lumbar interbody fusion: techniques, indications and comparison of interbody fusion options including PLIF, TLIF, MI-TLIF, OLIF/ATP, LLIF and ALIF. J Spine Surg 2015;1(1):2–18

6. Li JXJ, Phan K, Mobbs R. Oblique lumbar interbody fusion: technical aspects, operative outcomes, and complications. World Neurosurg 2017;98:113–123

7. de Kunder SL, van Kuijk SMJ, Rijkers K, et al. Transforaminal lumbar interbody fusion (TLIF) versus posterior lumbar interbody fusion (PLIF) in lumbar spondylolisthesis: a systematic review and meta-analysis. Spine J 2017;17(11):1712–1721

8. Murase S, Oshima Y, Takeshita Y, et al. Anterior cage dislodgement in posterior lumbar interbody fusion: a review of 12 patients. J Neurosurg Spine 2017;27(1):48–55

9. Ariyoshi D, Sano S, Kawamura N. Inferior vena cava injury caused by an anteriorly migrated cage resulting in ligation: case report. J Neurosurg Spine 2016;24(3):409–412

10. Pawar UM, Kundnani V, Nene A. Major vessel injury with cage migration: surgical complication in a case of spondylodiscitis. Spine 2010;35(14):E663–E666

11. Heary RF, Mummaneni PV. Editorial: vascular injury during spinal procedures. J Neurosurg Spine 2016;24(3):407–408, discussion 408

12. Quigley KJ, Alander DH, Bledsoe JG. An in vitro biomechanical investigation: variable positioning of leopard carbon fiber interbody cages. J Spinal Disord Tech 2008;21(6):442–447

13. Kwon BK, Berta S, Daffner SD, et al. Radiographic analysis of transforaminal lumbar interbody

fusion for the treatment of adult isthmic spondylolisthesis. J Spinal Disord Tech 2003;16(5): 469–476

14. Bono CM, Khandha A, Vadapalli S, Holekamp S, Goel VK, Garfin SR. Residual sagittal motion after lumbar fusion: a finite element analysis with implications on radiographic flexion-extension criteria. Spine 2007;32(4):417–422

15. Park SJ, Lee CS, Chung SS, Kang SS, Park HJ, Kim SH. The ideal cage position for achieving both indirect neural decompression and segmental angle restoration in lateral lumbar interbody fusion (LLIF). Clin Spine Surg 2017;30(6): E784–E790

16. Regev GJ, Haloman S, Chen L, et al. Incidence and prevention of intervertebral cage overhang with minimally invasive lateral approach fusions. Spine 2010;35(14):1406–1411

17. Kraiwattanapong C, Arnuntasupakul V, Kantawan R, et al. Malposition of cage in minimally invasive oblique lumbar interbody fusion. Case Rep Orthop 2018;2018:9142074

18. Park M-K, Kim K-T, Bang W-S, et al. Risk factors for cage migration and cage retropulsion following transforaminal lumbar interbody fusion. Spine J 2019;19(3):437–447

19. Pan F-M, Wang S-J, Yong Z-Y, Liu XM, Huang YF, Wu DS. Risk factors for cage retropulsion after lumbar interbody fusion surgery: series of cases and literature review. Int J Surg 2016;30:56–62

20. Lee D-Y, Park Y-J, Song S-Y, Jeong ST, Kim DH. Risk factors for posterior cage migration after lumbar interbody fusion surgery. Asian Spine J 2018;12(1):59–68

21. Aoki Y, Yamagata M, Nakajima F, et al. Examining risk factors for posterior migration of fusion cages following transforaminal lumbar interbody fusion: a possible limitation of unilateral pedicle screw fixation. J Neurosurg Spine 2010;13(3): 381–387

22. Kimura H, Shikata J, Odate S, Soeda T, Yamamura S. Risk factors for cage retropulsion after posterior lumbar interbody fusion: analysis of 1070 cases. Spine 2012;37(13):1164–1169

23. Bakhsheshian J, Khanna R, Choy W, et al. Incidence of graft extrusion following minimally invasive transforaminal lumbar interbody fusion. J Clin Neurosci 2016;24:88–93

24. Zaidi HA, Shah A, Kakarla UK. Transdural retrieval of a retropulsed lumbar interbody cage: technical case report. Asian J Neurosurg 2016;11(1):71

25. Nguyen H-V, Akbarnia BA, van Dam BE, et al. Anterior exposure of the spine for removal of lumbar interbody devices and implants. Spine 2006;31(21):2449–2453

26. Towers WS, Kurtom KH. Stand-alone LLIF lateral cage migration: a case report. Cureus 2015;7(10): e347

27. Chang C-W, Fu T-S, Chen W-J, Chen CW, Lai PL, Chen SH. Management of infected transforaminal lumbar interbody fusion cage in posterior degenerative lumbar spine surgery. World Neurosurg 2019;126:e330–e341

Chapter 12

Lumbar Interbody Fusion: Clinico-radiological Outcomes

12 Lumbar Interbody Fusion: Clinico-radiological Outcomes

Sajesh Menon

Introduction

Degeneration of the lumbar spine is a common ailment in the aging population and one of the most frequent causes of disability resulting in mechanical back pain, radicular and neurogenic claudication, reduced mobility, and poor quality of life. Surgical decompression is indicated in disabled patients, and often instrumentation and fusion of degenerative levels are employed to stabilize the painful motion segment, restore lordosis, and correct deformities if present. Many spinal fusion techniques have been developed since the initial description in the early 20th century and the commonly carried out surgical options in lumbar interbody fusion (LIF) include the traditional posterolateral intertransverse fusion (PLF), posterior LIF (PLIF), transforaminal LIF (TLIF), minimally invasive TLIF (MIS-TLIF), oblique LIF (OLIF), lateral LIF (LLIF), and anterior LIF (ALIF).

The clinico-radiological outcome studies have assumed a greater relevance with the advent of these new and minimally invasive surgeries in LIF. Understanding the clinico-radiological outcome is important for the use of a specific and relevant technique in the given lumbar spine disease. The outcome studies also help us in comparing the advantages/disadvantages of one technique over another.

Assessment of Functional Improvement

The clinical outcome measurement of any intervention is important to gauge the treatment effectiveness and efficiency. In LIF surgeries, the common clinical scales used for measurement of postoperative outcomes are quite standard in a majority of studies. In a meta-analysis on assessment of functional outcome scores used in lumbar surgery, Ghogawala et al recommend Oswestry Disability Index (ODI) as a dominant disease-specific outcome measure for assessment of clinical improvement. They also found Short Form-36 (SF-36) and the more recent SF-12 emerging as dominant general health outcome measures.[1] Hence, there is a need for a treating physician/surgeon to be familiar of these health-related quality of life (HRQL) scores.

Health-Related Quality of Life Scores

HRQL tools are a set of questionnaires that patients have to complete regarding what activities they can do, how often they can do them, and the level of difficulty they have in performing them. The reliability and validity of HQRL tools have been extensively studied[2,3] and are well established. In general, HRQL tools are classified as generic (SF-36, SF-12), condition specific (RMQ, ODI), and patient specific.[4]

Short Form Survey-36 and 12

SF-36 is the most commonly used questionnaire and its reliability in patients with low back pain has been extensively validated.[5] It has two components—the physical component summary score (PCS) and the mental component summary score (MCS). These components further have eight different health concepts including general health, physical functioning, role functioning, bodily pain, mental health, emotional functioning, vitality, and social functioning.[6] It is available in 12 languages and the standard version is based on 30-day recall. It is a self-administered questionnaire that takes 5 to 10 minutes for the patients to fill it up.

SF-12 has 12 questions (**Fig. 12.1**) to reduce the time needed (<5 minutes) to fill the questionnaire and has two components similar to SF-36. Even though it is valid and reliable,[7] it is

1. In general, would you say your health is:				
☐1 Excellent	☐2 Very good	☐3 Good	☐4 Fair	☐5 Poor

The following questions are about activities you might do during a typical day. Does <u>your health now limit you</u> in these activities? If so, how much?

	Yes, limited a lot	Yes, limited a little	No, not limited at all
2. Moderate activities such as moving a table, pushing a vacuum cleaner, bowling, or playing golf.	☐1	☐2	☐3
3. Climbing several flights of stairs.	☐1	☐2	☐3

During the <u>past 4 weeks</u>, have you had any of the following problems with your work or other regular daily activities <u>as a result of your physical health</u>?

	Yes	No
4. Accomplished less than you would like.	☐1	☐2
5. Were limited in the kind of work or other activities.	☐1	☐2

During the <u>past 4 weeks</u>, have you had any of the following problems with your work or other regular daily activities <u>as a result of any emotional problems</u> (such as feeling depressed or anxious)?

	Yes	No
6. Accomplished less than you would like.	☐1	☐2
7. Did work or activities less carefully than usual.	☐1	☐2

8. During the <u>past 4 weeks</u>, how much <u>did pain interfere</u> with your normal work (including work outside the home and housework)?

☐1 Not at all	☐2 A little bit	☐3 Moderately	☐4 Quite a bit	☐5 Extremely

These questions are about how you have been feeling during the <u>past 4 weeks</u>.
For each question, please give the one answer that comes closest to the way you have been feeling.

How much of the time during the <u>past 4 weeks</u>...

	All of the time	Most of the time	A good bit of the time	Some of the time	A little of the time	None of the time
9. Have you felt calm & peaceful?	☐1	☐2	☐3	☐4	☐5	☐6
10. Did you have a lot of energy?	☐1	☐2	☐3	☐4	☐5	☐6
11. Have you felt down-hearted and blue?	☐1	☐2	☐3	☐4	☐5	☐6

12. During the <u>past 4 weeks</u>, how much of the time has your <u>physical health or emotional problems</u> interfered with your social activities (like visiting friends, relatives, etc.)?

☐1 All of the time	☐2 Most of the time	☐3 Some of the time	☐4 A little of the time	☐5 None of the time

Fig. 12.1 Short Form Health Survey (SF-12).

limited only for group comparisons rather than individual decisions.[8]

Roland Morris Low Back Pain and Disability Questionnaire

The Roland Morris low back pain and disability questionnaire (RMQ) is a widely used disease-specific measure for low back pain. Its reliability, validity, and utility have been well established among these patients.[9,10] The tool consists of 24 questions related to pain and function (**Fig. 12.2**) with each item having a score of either 1 or 0. The RMQ takes 5 minutes to complete and only 1 minute to score. If, for example, preoperatively, a patient's score was 14 and at the postsurgery follow-up the score was 4, the patient has improved by 10 points and percentage of improvement is 71% ($10/14 \times 100$).

Oswestry Disability Index Scoring

The ODI score was developed in 1980s and since then there has been multiple modifications and all are in current use. The ODI questionnaires

Roland-Morris Low Back Pain and Disability Questionnaire (RMQ)

Instructions

Patient name: _____ File # _____ Date: _____

Please read instructions: When your back hurts, you may find it difficult to do some of the things you normally do. Mark only the sentences that describe you today.

☐ I stay at home most of the time because of my back.

☐ I change position frequently to try to get my back confortable.

☐ I walk more slowly than usual because of my back.

☐ Because of my back, I am not doing any jobs that I usually do around the house.

☐ Because of my back, I use a handrail to get upstairs.

☐ Because of my back, I lie down to rest more often.

☐ Because of my back, I have to hold on to something to get out of an easy chair.

☐ Because of my back, I try to get other people to do thins for me.

☐ I find it difficult to get out of a chair becuase of my back.

☐ My back is painful almost all of the time.

☐ I find it difficult to turn over in bed because of my back.

☐ My appetite is not ver good because of my back.

☐ I have trouble putting on my socks (or stockings) because of the pain in my back.

☐ I can only walk short distances because of my back pain.

☐ I sleep less well because of my back.

☐ Because of my back pain, I get dressed with the help of someone else.

☐ I sit down for most of the day because of my back.

☐ I avoid heavy jobs around the house because of my back.

☐ Because of my back pain, I am more irritable and bad tempered with people than usual.

☐ Because of my back, I go upstais more slowly than usual.

☐ I stay in bed most of the time because of my back.

Fig. 12.2 Roland Morris low back pain and disability questionnaire.

are disease specific, reliable, and valid.[2,11,12] This questionnaire is self-administered like others and takes 5 minutes to complete and ~1 minute for scoring. The 10 questions are framed in such a way that it measures the activities of daily living and pain with increasing degree of severity relating to a particular activity. These sections are scored from 0 to 5 points. The total raw score is added and multiplied by 2 to provide a percentage of disability[13] (**Fig. 12.3**)

Patient-Specific Measures

This measurement involves choosing any five activities/work specific to the patient that they find difficult to perform because of the disease.

These activities are then rated from 0 to 10 with 0 being "inability" to 10 being "full performance without any difficulty." This is highly patient specific and they are compared pre- and postoperatively. It takes 15 minutes to complete and involves active participation of the therapist or treating physician. It has been proved to be highly reliable and valid.[14,15]

Assessment of Radiological Outcomes

Radiological methods for the assessment of spinal fusion include standard radiography, dynamic radiography, radiostereometric

Owestry Low Back Pain Disability Questionnaire

Instructions

This questionnaire has been designed to give us information as to how your back of leg pain is affecting your ability to manage in everyday life. Please answer by cheking ONE box in each section for the statement which best applies to you. We realise you may consider that two or more statements in any one section apply but please just shade out the spot that indicates the statement which most clearly describes your problem.

Section 1 – Pain intensity
- ☐ I have no pain at the moment
- ☐ The pain is very mild at the moment
- ☐ The pain is moderate at the moment
- ☐ The pain is fairly severe at the moment
- ☐ The pain is very severe at the moment
- ☐ The pain is the worst imaginable at the moment

Section 2 – Personal care (washing, dressing etc)
- ☐ I can look after myself normally without causing extra pain
- ☐ I can look after myself normally but it causes extra pain
- ☐ It is painful to look after myself and I am slow and careful
- ☐ I need some help but manage most of my personal care
- ☐ I need help every day in most aspects of self-care
- ☐ I do not get dressed, I wash with difficulty and stay in bed

Section 3 – Lifting
- ☐ I can lift heavy weights without extra pain
- ☐ I can lift heavy weights but it gives extra pain
- ☐ Pain prevents me from lifting heavy weights off the floor, but I can manage if they are conveniently placed eg. on a table
- ☐ Pain prevents me from lifting heavy weights, but I can manage light to medium weights if they are conveniently positioned
- ☐ I can lift very light weights
- ☐ I cannot lift or carry enything at all

Section 4 – Walking
- ☐ Pain does not prevent me walking any distance
- ☐ Pain prevents me from walking more than 1 mile
- ☐ Pain prevents me from walking more than ½ mile
- ☐ Pain prevents me from walking more than 100 yards
- ☐ I can only walk using a stick or crutches
- ☐ I am in bed most of the time

Section 5 – Sitting
- ☐ I can sit in any chair as long as I like
- ☐ I can only sit in my favourite chair as long as I like
- ☐ Pain prevents me sitting more than one hour
- ☐ Pain prevents me from sitting more than 30 minutes
- ☐ Pain prevents me from sitting more than 10 minutes
- ☐ Pain prevents me from sitting at all

Section 6 – Standing
- ☐ I can stand as long as I want without extra pain
- ☐ I can stand as long as I want but it gives me extra pain
- ☐ Pain prevents me from standing for more than 1 hour
- ☐ Pain prevents me from standing for more than 30 minutes
- ☐ Pain prevents me from standing for more than 10 minutes
- ☐ Pain prevents me from standing at all

Section 7 – Sleeping
- ☐ My sleep is never disturbed by pain
- ☐ My sleep is occasionally disturbed by pain
- ☐ Because of pain I have less than 6 hours sleep
- ☐ Because of pain I have less than 4 hours sleep
- ☐ Because of pain I have less than 2 hours sleep
- ☐ Pain prevents me from sleeping at all

Section 8 – Sex life (if applicable)
- ☐ My sex life is normal and causes no extra pain
- ☐ My sex life is normal but causes some extra pain
- ☐ My sex life is nearly normal but is very painful
- ☐ My sex life is severely restricted by pain
- ☐ My sex life is nearly absent because of pain
- ☐ Pain prevents any sex life at all

Section 9 – Social life
- ☐ My social life is normal and gives me no extra pain
- ☐ Pain has no significant effect on my social life apart from limiting my more energetic interests eg, sport
- ☐ Pain has restricted my social life and I do not go out as often
- ☐ Pain has restricted my social life to my home
- ☐ I have no social life because of pain

Section 10 – Travelling
- ☐ I can travel anywhere without pain
- ☐ I can travel anywhere but it gives me extra pain
- ☐ Pain is bad but I manage journeys over two hours
- ☐ Pain restricts me to journeys of less than one hour
- ☐ Pain restricts me to short necessary journeys under 30 minutes
- ☐ Pain prevents me from travelling except to receive treatment

Fig. 12.3 Oswestry Disability Index scoring.

Interpretations of scores	
0% to 20%: minimal disability	The patient can cope with most living activities. Usually no treatment is indicated apart from advice on lifting sitting and exercise.
21% to 40%: moderate disability	The patients experiences more pain and difficulty with sitting, lifting and standing. Travel and social life are more difficult and they may be disabled from work. Personal care, sexual activity and sleeping are not grossly affected and the patient can usually be managed by conservative means.
41% to 60%: severe disability	Pain remains the main problem in this group but activities of daily living are affected. These patients require a detailed investigation.
61% to 80%: cripled	Back pain impinges on all aspects of the patient's life. Positive intervention is required
81% to 100%	These patients are either bed-bound or exaggerating their symptoms.

Fig. 12.3 *(Continued)* Oswestry Disability Index scoring.

analysis, computed tomography (CT), and magnetic resonance imaging (MRI). Radiological assessment is done postoperatively to confirm the correct position and the integrity of instrumentation, assess the progress of osseous fusion, detect suspected complications, and look for any new disease or disease progression. There is currently no reference standard for noninvasive imaging and evaluation of fusion. The modality and protocol used to image the postoperative spine depends on the site, clinical situation in question, and the type of instrumentation. The technical success of fusion is defined as the presence of bridging trabecular bone across fused vertebral bodies, facet joints, and transverse processes. The gold standard for determining this should be open exploration and direct examination of the fused segments.[16] However, this is certainly useful in the experimental setting and apart from revision cases, its practicality and usefulness in the clinical setting is very limited. Hence, the assessment of spinal fusion largely relies on noninvasive radiological methods. Though the radiographic feature of nonunion is primarily the graft resorption, other secondary features provide indirect assessment of nonunion. They are tabulated in **Box 12.1**.

The confirmation of fusion/pseudoarthrosis is not always easy and often complicated by anatomical differences, implant artifacts, presence of physiological motion at fused segments, and patient characteristic such as obesity, osteoporosis, etc.

Plain Radiography

Plain radiography has been the most commonly employed method to assess spinal fusion.

Box 12.1 Radiology features of nonunion

- Radiolucency around metalwork (increasing over time or persisting at 2 years)
- Lucency between cage and vertebral end plate
- Vacuum phenomenon
- Implant fracture
- Migration/subsidence of implant
- Loss of graft height
- Progressive deformity on loading

Advantages of using X-ray include easy availability, relatively low cost, ease of application, and relative safety for the patient. However, the reliability of this modality is questionable in detecting small voids associated with pseudoarthrosis, and it has limitations in demonstrating across coronal and sagittal planes especially in the thoracic and lumbar spine. Blumenthal and Gill[17] compared surgical exploration with plain radiographs to detect combined interbody and posterolateral fusion in the lumbar spine and they demonstrated only 69% overall agreement between the two methods. Kant et al[18] found that nearly one-quarter of those classified as fused on plain radiographs were in fact not fused on surgical exploration. Santos et al[19] demonstrated that plain radiographs identified only 4/15 nonunion that were identified on CT.

Functional Radiography

Functional or dynamic radiography was introduced to rectify some of the fallacies associated with plain radiographs. It is performed in an attempt to detect any movement within the fused motion segment. Presence of any motion across the fusion motion segment is considered as nonunion or pseudoarthrosis. However, a certain degree of movement within the fused segment has been observed on flexion-extension radiographs even in confirmed cases due to the inherent elasticity of bone. Hence, various motion threshold for allowable movement on dynamic radiographs in the lumbar spine have been described to define pseudoarthrosis.

According to the US Food and Drug Administration, a "stable bony union" is defined as having < 5 degree of movement on flexion-extension radiographs whereas Simmons et al[20] defined fusion as < 2 degree of movement. The Hutter method relies on superimposing the plain films in flexion and extension over one another to detect motion between the fused segments.[21] Using a finite element analysis model, Bono et al[22] demonstrated wide variation in residual flexion-extension motion depending on the type of fusion (interbody/intertransverse fusion).

There are many other studies that show lack of consensus on the allowable movement at a fused segment, which makes dynamic radiographs potentially unreliable.

Computed Tomography

The ability of modern CT scanners to take fine-cut slices of 0.5 to 1 mm, helical acquisition, multiplanar reconstruction, and implant artifact reduction, has a distinct advantage of assessing fusion. It can detail the bridging trabecular bone with resolution, which is indicative of arthrodesis.[23] Studies have shown that CT has 89% probability of correct demonstration of fusion in lumbar spine.[24] Regarding the intra- and interobserver reliability, CT is much superior to radiographs, and Carreon et al[25] proved that three-dimensional CT has considerably greater degree of interobserver and intraobserver agreement compared with anteroposterior and flexion/extension radiographs alone.

CT-based assessment of fusion both through a metallic cage and in the presence of bridging anterior or posterior bone, commonly referred as "sentinel sign," has been demonstrated to have only fair interobserver reliability.[26] Santos et al demonstrated that accuracy of using CT is 65% to detect fusion with a carbon fiber cage compared with 74 to 96% using radiographic methods.[27] They also introduced the concept

"locked pseudoarthrosis" to describe a non-union demonstrated within an interbody cage on CT. Based on this concept, Brantigan, Steffee, and Fraser introduced Brantigan–Steffee–Fraser (BSF) classification of interbody fusion success. According to this classification, a BSF-1 pseudoarthrosis is indicated by collapse of the construct, loss of disc height, vertebral slip, broken screws, and displacement of cage, resorption of bone graft, or visible lucency around periphery of graft or cage. BSF-2 represents locked pseudoarthrosis and BSF-3 defines radiographical fusion of bone bridging at least half the fusion area, with at least the density originally achieved at surgery.[28] Radiographical fusion through one cage (half of the fusion area) is considered to be mechanically a "solid fusion" even if there is lucency on the opposite side. Other major drawbacks of CT are the depth of radiation exposure to a patient. A single lumbar spine CT examination is equivalent to the radiation exposure from ~240 chest radiographs[29] and each exposure carries a 1 in 3,300 risk of inducing a fatal cancer. In view of these risks, it is recommended that use of CT should be employed judiciously and only in indicated cases.

Magnetic Resonance Imaging

MRI is an attractive alternate to CT due to the lack of ionizing radiation exposure, however, there is limited data on the use of MRI to assess spinal fusion postoperatively. In a study Kröner et al[30] demonstrated successful assessment of bony bridging in 49 PLIF patients with a carbon fiber cage by 1T MRI using specific sequence protocols. The authors reported that metal artifacts from posterior instrumentation exerted minimal influence than expected in evaluating the success of fusion. In general, metallic artifacts can make assessment of fusion on MRI difficult, particularly in the posterolateral region adjacent to rods and screws or in the presence of a metallic interbody cage. Interestingly, as the magnet strength increases, so does susceptibility to metallic artifact and hence the lower-strength magnets are superior for assessing fusion than the latest 3T scanners. Though MRI does have a distinct advantage in postoperative evaluation of the neural elements and other possible causes of persistent/recurrent symptoms following spinal fusion, further work is needed to determine its role in assessing the adequacy of fusion.

Nuclear Medicine

Bone scintigraphy can be performed to assess fusion in difficult cases and the fused segment should be nonactive or cold after 6 to 12 months. A study has shown a higher accuracy in Single-photon Emission CT (SPECT)/CT versus planar SPECT which utilizes additional CT spatial correlation in diagnosing pathologies in patients with previous spinal surgery. There is also increased specificity using SPECT/CT for detection of nonunion of interbody devices compared with CT alone.[31]

Hence, CT scans (fine-cut axial and multiplanar reconstruction) appear to be the most effective noninvasive method of determining fusion status even in the presence of spinal instrumentation. Other radiographic techniques have shown some utility as well, such as radioisotope scans have good sensitivity to detect pseudoarthrosis and can be combined with CT to enhance the effectiveness of each modality.

Fusion Rates of Different Lumbar Fusion Techniques

The fusion rates in lumbar spine surgery can vary according to the technique/approach. However, studies on LIF show that there is no solid evidence to show the superiority of one fusion method over the other in terms of functional outcomes. In the study reported by Christensen et al,[32] the PLF group had a fusion rate of 80% and that of PLIF and ALIF were 92 and 82%, respectively. Kim et al[33] compared the clinical outcomes of three posterior fusion methods: PLF, PLIF, and circumferential fusion. All three groups showed high union rates at the last follow-up: 92% in PLF group, 95% in PLIF group, and 93% for the circumferential group. They clearly demonstrated that there was no significant difference between the union rates. Inamdar et al[34] recommended PLF over PLIF because of the simplicity of the procedure, lower complication rate, and good clinical and radiological outcomes, even though the

fusion rates were 100% in both groups. In the study reported by Hallett et al,[35] PLF had solid fusion rates in more than 90% of stabilized patients; however the fusion rates of TLIF were less clearly demonstrable compared with PLF. There was no significant difference between the groups in terms of the functional results. However, Yan et al[36] and Zhuo et al[37] reported 100% radiographic fusion rates in both PLIF and TLIF. Audat et al[38] and Sakeb et al[39] reported no significant differences in radiographic fusion rates between PLIF and TLIF.

A systematic review by Lee et al[40] stated no difference in fusion rates between ALIF plus posterior transpedicular instrumentation and circumferential fusion versus PLIF and circumferential fusion. However, they concluded that a general statement could not be made because of the scarcity of data, heterogeneity of the trials included, and some methodological defects.

Mummaneni et al,[41] in a meta-analysis study on interbody techniques for lumbar fusion, found that there is no conclusive evidence supporting better clinical or radiographic outcomes based on the technique. They also concluded that no general recommendation can, therefore, be made regarding the technique that should be used to achieve interbody fusion. In short, although numerous studies on spinal fusion have been conducted, their outcomes are so inconsistent that it is difficult to determine which approach provides the highest fusion rate or better clinical outcome.

Clinical Relevance of Pseudoarthrosis

Radiological demonstration of a solid fusion across the stabilized segments is the primary goal of every lumbar fusion procedure performed to treat lumbar degenerative disease. Theoretically, patients who achieve a solid fusion would be expected to have better clinical outcomes compared with pseudoarthrosis. However, many studies describe the controversial relationship between clinical outcome and radiological outcome,[42] and many patients with demonstrable successful fusion on radiological assessment may not show clinical success and vice versa.

Clinical success often encompasses other factors such as pain reduction, improved function, and patient satisfaction. Ultimately, careful patient selection and realistic clinical outcome measures such as visual analog score, ODI, Japanese Orthopaedic Association score, SF-36 scores may be more important than the radiological outcome of surgery in determining a successful outcome. Radiological assessment has the ability to demonstrate a solid arthrodesis or a pseudoarthrosis. The demonstration of nonunion is more critical for patients with persistent or recurrent symptoms postoperatively. Revision surgery should be considered in such patients with demonstrable pseudoarthrosis and it is rarely done to manage asymptomatic pseudarthrosis.

Summary

The primary goal of LIF is to achieve a solid arthrodesis. Assessment of functional outcome following lumbar spinal fusion is essential for comparing the effectiveness of surgical treatments. When assessing functional outcome of these patients, a reliable, valid, and responsive outcome measure such as the ODI should be used. The SF-36 and the SF-12 also have emerged as dominant measures of general HRQL.

CT alone or in combination with SPECT appears to have greater sensitivity when assessing for successful fusion. However, plane radiography, dynamic radiography, and MRI all appear to have a role in the diagnostic pathway of fusion at differing stages of the postoperative period. At times, combination of these modalities may be required in difficult cases. Although a definitive cause and effect relationship has not been demonstrated, there is moderate evidence that demonstrates a positive association between radiographical presence of fusion and improved clinical outcomes. Hence, it is recommended that strategies intended to enhance the potential for radiographical fusion should be considered when performing a lumbar instrumentation for degenerative spine disease.

References

1. Ghogawala Z, Resnick DK, Watters WC III, et al. Guideline update for the performance of fusion procedures for degenerative disease of the lumbar spine. Part 2: assessment of functional outcome following lumbar fusion. J Neurosurg Spine 2014;21(1):7–13
2. Fairbank JC, Couper J, Davies JB, O'Brien JP. The Oswestry low back pain disability questionnaire. Physiotherapy 1980;66(8):271–273
3. Gatchel RJ, Polatin PB, Mayer TG, Robinson R, Dersh J. Use of the SF-36 Health Status Survey with a chronically disabled back pain syndrome: strengths and limitations. J Occup Rehabil 1998;8:237–246
4. Resnik L, Dobrzykowski E. Guide to outcomes measurement for patients with low back pain syndromes. J Orthop Sports Phys Ther 2003;33(6):307–316, discussion 317–318
5. Taylor SJ, Taylor AE, Foy MA, Fogg AJ. Responsiveness of common outcome measures for patients with low back pain. Spine 1999;24(17):1805–1812
6. Ware JE Jr, Snow KK, Kosinski M, Gandek B. SF-36 Health Survey: Manual and Interpretation Guide. Boston, MA: Health Insititute, New England Medical Center; 1993
7. Ware J Jr, Kosinski M, Keller SDA. A 12-Item Short-Form Health Survey: construction of scales and preliminary tests of reliability and validity. Med Care 1996;34(3):220–233
8. Riddle DL, Lee KT, Stratford PW. Use of SF-36 and SF-12 health status measures: a quantitative comparison for groups versus individual patients. Med Care 2001;39(8):867–878
9. Stratford PW, Binkley JM. Applying the results of self-report measures to individual patients: an example using the Roland-Morris Questionnaire. J Orthop Sports Phys Ther 1999;29(4):232–239
10. Stratford PW, Binkley J, Solomon P, Finch E, Gill C, Moreland J. Defining the minimum level of detectable change for the Roland-Morris Questionnaire. Phys Ther 1996;76(4):359–365, discussion 366–368
11. Beurskens AJ, de Vet HC, Köke AJ. Responsiveness of functional status in low back pain: a comparison of different instruments. Pain 1996;65(1):71–76
12. Leclaire R, Blier F, Fortin L, Proulx R. A cross-sectional study comparing the Oswestry and Roland-Morris Functional Disability scales in two populations of patients with low back pain of different levels of severity. Spine 1997;22(1):68–71
13. Fairbank JC, Pynsent PB. The Oswestry Disability Index. Spine 2000;25(22):2940–2952, discussion 2952
14. Beurskens AJ, de Vet HC, Köke AJ, et al. A patient-specific approach for measuring functional status in low back pain. J Manipulative Physiol Ther 1999;22(3):144–148
15. Stratford P, Gill C, Westaway MD. Assessing disability and change on individual patients: a

report of a patient specific measure. Physiother Can 1995;47:258–263

16. Cook SD, Patron LP, Christakis PM, Bailey KJ, Banta C, Glazer PA. Comparison of methods for determining the presence and extent of anterior lumbar interbody fusion. Spine 2004;29(10): 1118–1123

17. Blumenthal SL, Gill K. Can lumbar spine radiographs accurately determine fusion in postoperative patients? Correlation of routine radiographs with a second surgical look at lumbar fusions. Spine 1993;18(9):1186–1189

18. Kant AP, Daum WJ, Dean SM, Uchida T. Evaluation of lumbar spine fusion. Plain radiographs versus direct surgical exploration and observation. Spine 1995;20(21):2313–2317

19. Santos ER, Goss DG, Morcom RK, Fraser RD. Radiologic assessment of interbody fusion using carbon fiber cages. Spine 2003;28(10):997–1001

20. Simmons JW, Andersson GB, Russell GS, Hadjipavlou AG. A prospective study of 342 patients using transpedicular fixation instrumentation for lumbosacral spine arthrodesis. J Spinal Disord 1998;11(5):367–374

21. Hutter CG. Posterior intervertebral body fusion. A 25-year study. Clin Orthop Relat Res 1983;(179): 86–96

22. Bono CM, Khandha A, Vadapalli S, Holekamp S, Goel VK, Garfin SR. Residual sagittal motion after lumbar fusion: a finite element analysis with implications on radiographic flexion-extension criteria. Spine 2007;32(4):417–422

23. Kataoka ML, Hochman MG, Rodriguez EK, Lin PJ, Kubo S, Raptopolous VD; EK. A review of factors that affect artifact from metallic hardware on multi-row detector computed tomography. Curr Probl Diagn Radiol 2010;39(4):125–136

24. Carreon LY, Djurasovic M, Glassman SD, Sailer P. Diagnostic accuracy and reliability of fine-cut CT scans with reconstructions to determine the status of an instrumented posterolateral fusion with surgical exploration as reference standard. Spine 2007;32(8):892–895

25. Carreon LY, Glassman SD, Djurasovic M. Reliability and agreement between fine-cut CT scans and plain radiography in the evaluation of posterolateral fusions. Spine J 2007;7(1):39–43

26. Carreon LY, Glassman SD, Schwender JD, Subach BR, Gornet MF, Ohno S. Reliability and accuracy of fine-cut computed tomography scans to determine the status of anterior interbody fusions with metallic cages. Spine J 2008;8(6):998–1002

27. McAfee PC, Boden SD, Brantigan JW, et al. Symposium: a critical discrepancy—a criteria of successful arthrodesis following interbody spinal fusions. Spine 2001;26(3):320–334

28. Fogel GR, Toohey JS, Neidre A, Brantigan JW. Fusion assessment of posterior lumbar interbody fusion using radiolucent cages: X-ray films and helical computed tomography scans compared with surgical exploration of fusion. Spine J 2008; 8(4):570–577

29. Biswas D, Bible JE, Bohan M, Simpson AK, Whang PG, Grauer JN. Radiation exposure from musculoskeletal computerized tomographic scans. J Bone Joint Surg Am 2009;91(8):1882–1889

30. Kröner AH, Eyb R, Lange A, Lomoschitz K, Mahdi T, Engel A. Magnetic resonance imaging evaluation of posterior lumbar interbody fusion. Spine 2006; 31(12):1365–1371

31. Rager O, Schaller K, Payer M, Tchernin D, Ratib O, Tessitore E. SPECT/CT in differentiation of pseudarthrosis from other causes of back pain in lumbar spinal fusion: report on 10 consecutive cases. Clin Nucl Med 2012;37(4):339–343

32. Christensen FB, Hansen ES, Eiskjaer SP, et al. Circumferential lumbar spinal fusion with Brantigan cage versus posterolateral fusion with titanium Cotrel-Dubousset instrumentation: a prospective, randomized clinical study of 146 patients. Spine 2002;27(23):2674–2683

33. Kim KT, Lee SH, Lee YH, Bae SC, Suk KS. Clinical outcomes of 3 fusion methods through the posterior approach in the lumbar spine. Spine 2006;31(12):1351–1357, discussion 1358

34. Inamdar DN, Alagappan M, Shyam L, Devadoss S, Devadoss A. Posterior lumbar interbody fusion versus intertransverse fusion in the treatment of lumbar spondylolisthesis. J Orthop Surg (Hong Kong) 2006;14(1):21–26

35. Hallett A, Huntley JS, Gibson JN. Foraminal stenosis and single-level degenerative disc disease: a randomized controlled trial comparing decompression with decompression and instrumented fusion. Spine 2007;32(13):1375–1380

36. Yan DL, Li J, Gao LB, Soo CL. Comparative study on two different methods of lumbar interbody fusion with pedicle screw fixation for the treatment of spondylolisthesis. Zhonghua Wai Ke Za Zhi 2008;46(7):497–500

37. Zhuo X, Hu J, Li B, Sun H, Chen Y, Hu Z. Comparative study of treating recurrent lumbar disc protrusion by three different surgical procedures. Zhongguo Xiu Fu Chong Jian Wai Ke Za Zhi 2009;23(12):1422–1426

38. Audat Z, Moutasem O, Yousef K, Mohammad B. Comparison of clinical and radiological results of posterolateral fusion, posterior lumbar interbody fusion and transforaminal lumbar interbody fusion techniques in the treatment of degenerative lumbar spine. Singapore Med J 2012; 53(3):183–187

39. Sakeb N, Ahsan K. Comparison of the early results of transforaminal lumbar interbody fusion and posterior lumbar interbody fusion in symptomatic lumbar instability. Indian J Orthop 2013; 47:255–263

40. Lee CS, Hwang CJ, Lee DH, Kim YT, Lee HS. Fusion rates of instrumented lumbar spinal arthrodesis according to surgical approach: a systematic review of randomized trials. Clin Orthop Surg 2011;3:39–47

41. Mummaneni PV, Dhall SS, Eck JC, et al. Guideline update for the performance of fusion procedures for degenerative disease of the lumbar spine. Part 11: interbody techniques for lumbar fusion. J Neurosurg Spine 2014;21(1):67–74

42. Tuli SK, Chen P, Eichler ME, Woodard EJ. Reliability of radiologic assessment of fusion: cervical fibular allograft model. Spine 2004;29(8):856–860

Chapter 13

Current Literature Evidence for Lumbar Interbody Fusion

13 Current Literature Evidence for Lumbar Interbody Fusion

Arvind Bhave, Veeramani Preethish-Kumar

Introduction

Lumbar interbody fusion (LIF) is a well-established treatment for disorders affecting the lumbar spine as a result of several etiologies. Degeneration is the most prevalent pathology which affects the disc and the facet joints and may produce spondylolisthesis causing significant impairment of quality of life and higher pain scores. Patients who do not respond to conservative management require surgical intervention such as LIF. Various fusion methods such as anterior lumbar interbody fusion (ALIF), lateral lumbar interbody fusion (XLIF/LLIF), transforaminal lumbar interbody fusion (TLIF), and posterior lumbar interbody fusion (PLIF) exist based on the approach adapted to reach the spine.[1] The record of LIF dates back to Berthold Hadra, who performed the first instrumented spinal fusion procedure in 1891 Austin, TX. Later, Briggs promoted PLIF in 1944 and Jorgen Harms started TLIF in 1982.[2,3,4] The LIF technique has gained considerable refinement in recent years, and the relevant evidence regarding the appropriate fusion method is increasing as numerous studies are being conducted and published every year. Unfortunately, when cumulative evidence are taken together, it fails to definitively support one approach over another.

Multiple meta-analysis studies are done comparing the different LIF methods. For instance, in patients with degenerative lumbar spinal diseases, studies have compared open TLIF with minimally invasive TLIF, ALIF with TLIF, ALIF with posterior pedicle screw fixation (PPF) with standalone posterior approaches, etc. The predominant search databases used in all these studies include Cochrane Library database (including the Cochrane Central Register of Controlled Trials), PubMed (including MEDLINE), and various other sources extending from the date of inception to the commencement of analysis. The "levels of evidence" are an important component for practicing evidence-based medicine (**Table 13.1**).

Understanding this hierarchy and why levels are assigned to publications helps the reader to prioritize information. This does not mean level 4 evidence should be ignored and all level 1 evidence should be accepted as fact. These evidences act as a good guiding tool and majority of systematic reviews/meta-analyses contemplated in this chapter consider studies with level 1 to 4 evidence, however with caution, when interpreting these results. Universally, the primary outcomes analyzed in LIF studies are fusion rates, total blood loss during surgery, length of hospital stay, operation time, complication rates, fluoroscopic time, visual analog score (VAS), numeric rating scale (NRS),

Table 13.1 Levels of evidence for therapeutic studies

Level	Type of evidence
1A	Systematic review (with homogeneity) of RCTs
1B	Individual RCT (with narrow confidence intervals)
1C	All or none study
2A	Systematic review (with homogeneity) of cohort studies
2B	Individual cohort study (including low-quality RCT, for example, < 80% follow-up)
2C	"Outcomes" research; ecological studies
3A	Systematic review (with homogeneity) of case-control studies
3B	Individual case-control study
4	Case series (and poor-quality cohort) and case-control study
5	Expert opinion without explicit critical appraisal or based on physiology bench research or "first principles"

Abbreviation: RCT, randomized controlled trial.
Source: Centre for Evidence-Based Medicine, http://www.cebm.net.

Short Form-36 (SF-36), Japanese Orthopaedic Association (JOA) back pain evaluation, and Oswestry Disability Index (ODI). The approach in this chapter is to compile the current literature evidence for choosing the ideal LIF method for various disease conditions and also to establish the advantage of one method over another.

Indications for Lumbar Interbody Fusion: Anterior/Posterior/Lateral

The advent of new instruments and implants combined with latest technological advances has expanded the spectrum of "indications for performing LIF" in the past decade.[5]

The current indications for LIF are as formulated in **Box 13.1**.

Current Evidence to Support Fusion Over Decompression Alone

The latest study is by Koenig S et al, and they did a meta-analysis of evidence level I to IV studies from 1996 comparing decompression alone and decompression plus fusion in the treatment of degenerative spondylolisthesis (DS).[6] The number of cases that met the inclusion criteria in the decompression cohort was 12 (591 cases), and 13 cases (465 cases) in the fusion cohort. There was significant decrement in pain (legs and lower back), and SF-36 (physical, mental component) showed better patient clinical outcomes in both the cohorts.

Box 13.1 Indications for Lumbar Interbody Fusion

- Spondylolisthesis (usually grade I or II)
- Degenerative disc disease (DDD) causing discogenic low back pain (with or without radiculopathy)
- Recurrent lumbar disc herniation inducing significant mechanical back pain
- Postdiscectomy collapse with neural foraminal stenosis and secondary radiculopathy
- Greater recurrent or > 3 times recurrent lumbar disc herniation with or without pain
- Pseudoarthrosis
- Postlaminectomy kyphosis
- Lumbar coronal and/or sagittal deformities

In the decompression cohort, the values of 29.7 and 35.5 (physical and mental), improved to 41.2 and 48.5 points, respectively. In the fusion cohort, 28.4 and 39.3 points improved to 41.5 and 48.3 points, respectively. The complication rate was 5.8% (95% CI 1.7–2.1) in the decompression cohort and 8.3% (95% CI 5.5–11.6) in the decompression plus fusion cohort. The rate of resurgery was higher in the decompression cohort (8.5%) compared with the decompression plus fusion cohort (4.9%). The majority in the decompression group was older patients with a higher percentage of leg pain and in case of younger patients, additional fusion was performed. A recent study by Chan AK et al compared the 24-month patient-reported outcomes after minimally invasive surgery (MIS)-TLIF and MIS decompression in lumbar DS. Of 608 patients, MIS-TLIF was associated with a lower reoperation rate and superior outcomes in disability, back pain, and patient satisfaction compared with MIS decompression alone.[7]

These studies clearly represent a changing trend toward interbody fusion compared with decompression alone in the recent times mainly due to the better postoperative outcomes and especially with the adaptability for MIS.

Evidences to Show Advantage of Anterior and Lateral Procedures

The three most widely used anterior/lateral LIF procedures include ALIF, transpsoas LLIF, and a prepsoas or anterior to the psoas oblique lumbar interbody fusion (OLIF). The primary surgical goal of any anterior procedure is to implant the largest possible interbody graft within the confines of the surgical exposure to facilitate fusion rates, maximize the segmental lordosis (SL), and provide indirect neural decompression. This is achieved by expansion of bony neural foramen, distraction of ligamentous stenosis occurring at the central canal, distributing the load across the instrumented vertebra, and in addition providing sagittal balance correction.[8] ALIF has efficient and direct access to reconstruct anterior column. It avoids injury to paraspinal musculature and their denervation, particularly when done as a stand-alone procedure or in combination with percutaneous posterior instrumentation.

A comprehensive meta-analysis of the published data from 2010 to 2019 by Cho et al, evaluating outcome measures such as lumbar lordosis (LL), SL, slip rate, disc height (DH), VAS score, and ODI, compared ALIF/LLIF with PPF against TLIF/PLIF in DS (**Table 13.2**). Despite comparable postoperative outcomes between the two groups, the anterior procedures were superior to posterior ones in terms of restoring the LL, SL, and DH.[9] Another meta-analysis by Teng et al, comparing four different approaches (ALIF, LLIF, PLIF, and TLIF), found similar fusion rates irrespective of the procedure. However, ALIF had superior radiological outcomes and better restoration of postoperative DH and SL. The complication rates were similar between anterior and posterior approaches.[10] A systematic review by Keorochana et al, comparing MIS-TLIF with MIS-LLIF in degenerative lumbar disease, used ODI, VAS, and postoperative complications as outcome measures. A total of 9,506 patients (5,728 MIS-TLIF and 3,778 MIS-LLIF group) were compared and found that the fusion rate was not significantly different between the two techniques.[11]

Thus, anterior LIF procedures overall indicate a comparable fusion rate to posterior LIF procedures and have an advantage of restoring the near normal lumbar spine anatomy. Since ALIF allows for preservation of the posterior ligaments and soft tissue, the likelihood of adjacent segment degeneration (ASD) is less; although, here have been no consistent findings in the literature substantiating this claim. ALIF has its own shortcomings such as retraction of iliac vessels at L4–L5 level that may lead to increased vascular injury or thrombosis with incidence rate of 0 to 18.2%.[12,13] The handling of the hypogastric plexus can cause neural injury with retrograde ejaculation (RE) in males. Certain reports suggest the risk to be as low as less than 1% whereas others report it up to 45%.[14] A prospective study by Sasso et al found that transperitoneal ALIF approach has 10 times greater chance of RE than the retroperitoneal approach.[15] The use of the monopolar cautery should be minimized and bipolar cautery should be preferable.[16] In addition, ALIF is also associated with abdominal hernias. When combined with posterior fixation it involves additional cost and surgery.[14,15] Complications of LLIF include urinary retention, tibialis anterior

Table 13.2 Compilation of meta-analysis and systematic reviews on comparison of anterior/lateral lumbar interbody fusion procedures with other approaches

Comparison	Author	Inclusion period (y)	Number of studies	Outcome measures	Results
Decompression alone vs. with fusion	Koenig et al	21	25	Blood loss, VAS, ODI, SF-36, JOA, NRS	VAS and SF-36 (physical, mental component) improved in both the groups. Rate of resurgery was higher in decompression cohort (8.5%) compared with fusion (4.9%)
ALIF/LLIF with PPF vs. TLIF/PLIF	Cho et al	10	8	LL, SL, slip rate, DH, VAS, ODI, fusion rate	Comparable postoperative outcomes between two groups. Anterior procedures had good restoration of LL, SL, and DH
ALIF vs. PLIF vs. TLIF vs. LLIF	Teng et al	Inception - 2015	40	LL, SL, DH, VAS, ODI, operative outcomes, fusion rate, complications	Similar fusion and complication rates among all procedures. ALIF had superior radiological outcomes and better restoration of DH and SL
MIS-TLIF vs. MIS-LLIF	Keorochana et al	Inception - 2016	58	VAS, ODI, operative outcomes, fusion rate	Fusion rates and postoperative outcomes not significantly different between the two techniques

Abbreviations: ALIF, anterior lumbar interbody fusion; DH, disc height; JOA, Japanese Orthopaedic Association score; LL, lumbar lordosis; LLIF, lateral lumbar interbody fusion; NRS, Numeric Rating Scale; ODI, Oswestry Disability Index; PLIF, posterior lumbar interbody fusion; PPF, posterior pedicle screw fixation; SF-36, Short Form-36; SL, segmental lordosis; TLIF, transforaminal lumbar interbody fusion; VAS, visual analog score.

weakness, and transient sensory deficits. The best available current literature demonstrates 30 to 40% of patients having postoperative deficits, primarily of the proximal leg. However, permanent symptoms are less common, affecting 4 to 5% of cases.[17] Vascular injuries are also less frequent compared with ALIF. Visceral injuries, pneumothorax, and diaphragm injuries are reported at times.

Evidence and Comparison of Posterior LIF Procedures

The major posterior approaches include PLIF and TLIF surgery. PLIF and TLIF provide good outcomes for any lumbar spine disease. However, TLIF has replaced PLIF due to its advantages such as higher rates of fusion, minimal complications, and similar postoperative outcomes.[18] In 2003, Foley et al[19] demonstrated that MIS-TLIF has even less perioperative complications than traditional open TLIF. Fujimori et al compared the clinical and radiological outcomes of prospective cohort of TLIF (24 cases) and PLIF cases (32 cases) in DS. The fusion rate was better in TLIF (96%) as opposed to PLIF (84%) and in addition the DH was better restored in TLIF group. ODI improvement and LL were similar in both the groups.[20]

There are multiple meta-analyses available in literature comparing the PLIF and TLIF with other lateral/anterior procedures and MIS-TLIF over open TLIF (**Table 13.3**). de Kunder et al did a meta-analysis to compare the effectiveness of TLIF and PLIF in reducing disability and rate of intra- and postoperative complications in patients with DS. TLIF was better in terms of complication rate, blood loss, and operation duration. Clinical outcomes were comparable, with a slightly lower postoperative ODI score for TLIF.[4] Another study by Zhang et al compared the perioperative results and complications associated with PLIF and TLIF, and collected evidence for choosing the better fusion method. They found that PLIF had a higher complication rate and TLIF reduced the rate of durotomy. No statistical difference was found between the two groups with regards to clinical satisfaction, blood loss, vertebral root injury, graft malposition, infection, or the rate

of radiographical fusion.[21] However, PLIF has its own limitations as the procedure involves retraction of the neural tissue for cage and graft insertion along with epidural bleeding. To overcome this, TLIF was introduced which has less perioperative complications and less bleeding. In addition, TLIF can also be safely administered above L3 level. Lee et al concluded that 10% of patients would undergo additional surgery for treating ASD within 10 years after index posterior lumbar fusion. They showed PLIF showing higher incidence of ASD and age > 60 years being independent risk factor.[22]

Comparison of MIS-TLIF Over Open TLIF and Other LIF Procedures

Xie et al performed meta-analysis of prospective and retrospective studies that compared MIS-TLIF with open TLIF. They found that MIS-TLIF was associated with a significant decrease in VAS score, ODI index, and blood loss along with early ambulation and shorter hospital stay compared with open TLIF. However, there were no significant differences in the fusion rate, complication rate, operation time, or need for resurgery.[23] Qin et al compared the clinical efficacy and safety between MIS-TLIF and open TLIF in treatment of single-level DS by systematic review and meta-analysis. MIS-TLIF was more efficacious and safe technique with reduced tissue trauma, quicker postoperative recovery, and better long-term functional outcomes.[24] A similar conclusion was obtained by meta-analysis of seven RCTs proving MIS-TLIF has less blood loss than open TLIF. However, in their study there was no significant difference in the length of hospital stay, postoperative VAS, and ODI.[25] Even in the obese patients MIS-TLIF was found superior to open TLIF.[26] In case of choosing an ideal LIF procedure for degenerative disc disease (DDD), a network meta-analysis of prospective studies comparing PLIF (open and MIS), TLIF (open and MIS), and ALIF showed that MIS-PLIF resulted in lower pain scores than open TLIF/open PLIF. MIS-PLIF also had low ODI score than open TLIF/open PLIF/ALIF. They concluded that MIS-PLIF may be a better procedure for DDD and open TLIF may not be recommended.[27]

Table 13.3 Compilation of meta-analysis and systematic reviews on comparison of posterior lumbar interbody fusion procedures

Comparison	Author	Inclusion period	Number of studies	Outcome measures	Results
PLIF vs. TLIF	Zhang et al	Inception - 2013	7	Operative outcomes, fusion rate, blood loss, complications	PLIF has high complication rate. No difference between two groups in clinical satisfaction, blood loss, root injury, graft malposition, infection, or fusion
PLIF vs. TLIF	de Kunder et al	Inception - 2016	192	VAS, ODI, complications, operative outcomes	TLIF has less complication rate, blood loss, and duration of surgery. Comparable clinical outcomes between groups
Open TLIF vs. MIS-TLIF	Xie et al	Inception - 2015	24	VAS, ODI, operative outcomes, fusion rate, blood loss, complications	MIS-TLIF has significant decrease in VAS, ODI, and blood loss; early ambulation and short hospital stay. No significant difference in fusion/complication rate, operation time/need for resurgery
Open TLIF vs. MIS-TLIF	Li et al	Inception - 2018	7	VAS, ODI, operative outcomes	MIS-TLIF has less blood loss. No significant difference in the length of hospital stay, postoperative VAS, and ODI
Open TLIF vs. MIS-TLIF	Qin et al	2010–2018	6	VAS, ODI, operative outcomes, fusion rate, complications, length of hospitalization, resurgery	MIS-TLIF is more efficacious and safe with less tissue trauma, quicker recovery, better long-term functional outcomes
Open TLIF vs. MIS-TLIF in obese individuals	Xie et al	Inception - 2017	7	VAS, ODI, operative outcomes, complications, length of hospitalization	MIS-TLIF is superior to open TLIF
PLIF (open and MIS) vs. TLIF (open and MIS) vs. ALIF in DDD	Lin EY	Inception - 2018	8	VAS, ODI, operative outcomes	MIS-PLIF has lower pain scores than open TLIF/PLIF and better ODI than open TLIF/open PLIF/ALIF

Abbreviations: ALIF, anterior lumbar interbody fusion; DDD, degenerative disc disease; DH, disc height; JOA, Japanese Orthopaedic Association score; LL, lumbar lordosis; MIS, minimally invasive surgery; NRS, Numeric Rating Scale; ODI, Oswestry Disability Index; PLIF, posterior lumbar interbody fusion; SF-36, Short Form-36; SL, segmental lordosis; TLIF, transforaminal lumbar interbody fusion; VAS, visual analog score.

Recommendation on the Appropriate Approach Required by Demonstration of Case-Based Scenarios Compiled through Literature Evidence

L4–L5 spondylolisthesis, disc prolapse, facetal hypertrophy, and preserved intervertebral DH. The ideal method would be TLIF and the choice of performing it as open or MIS should be based on the surgeon's expertise (**Fig. 13.1**). However, MIS-TLIF is preferred over open TLIF due to the better postoperative outcomes as discussed.[23,24,25]

Case 1

A 45-year-old female with unilateral L5 radiculopathy (VAS: 7/10) presents with secondary

Case 2

A 57-year-old patient presents with weakness of bilateral ankle dorsiflexion and neurogenic

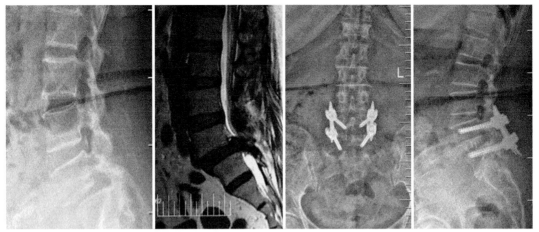

Fig. 13.1 L4–L5 spondylolisthesis managed with minimally invasive surgery transforaminal lumbar interbody fusion.

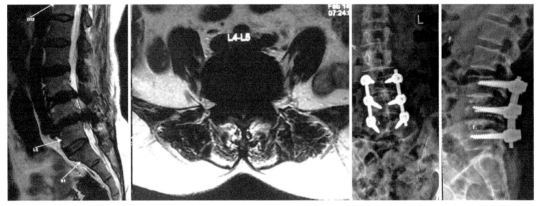

Fig. 13.2 L3–L5 lumbar canal stenosis with neurological deficits managed with open posterior interbody fusion.

claudication with magnetic resonance imaging (MRI) showing L3–L4 and L4–L5 lumbar canal stenosis, significant facetal hypertrophy, and preserved DH (**Fig. 13.2**). The surgery performed would be a two-level TLIF/PLIF as the DH is already better and there is the need to achieve a good decompression of the neural canal.[4]

Case 3

A 45-year-old female presents with significant back pain (VAS: 4/10), radicular pain in the distribution of L3 root with MRI showing L3–L4 DDD with instability, vacuum phenomenon, and significantly reduced disc space. This is an ideal case for anterior procedure, such as OLIF/ALIF, as it helps to increase the intervertebral DH and indirect foraminal decompression, and achieve desirable fusion (**Fig. 13.3**).[8–10]

Case 4

A 78-year-old patient presenting with back pain (VAS: 7/10) and neurogenic claudication for 100 m is diagnosed for degenerative lumbar scoliosis and flat back deformity from L2–S1 level. The patient will be benefitted by multilevel ALIF/OLIF and augmentation with PPF (**Fig. 13.4**). This procedure will be the treatment of choice for obtaining a better spinal balance in addition to neural decompression.[8]

Conclusion

In conclusion, it is evident that LIF, irrespective of the type of approach, remains an effective treatment option for a range of spinal disorders. Limited evidence is available for comparison of

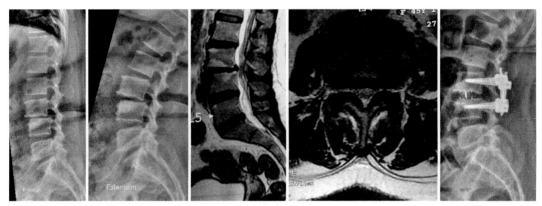

Fig. 13.3 L3–L4 degenerative disc disease with exiting nerve root pathology treated by oblique lumbar interbody fusion.

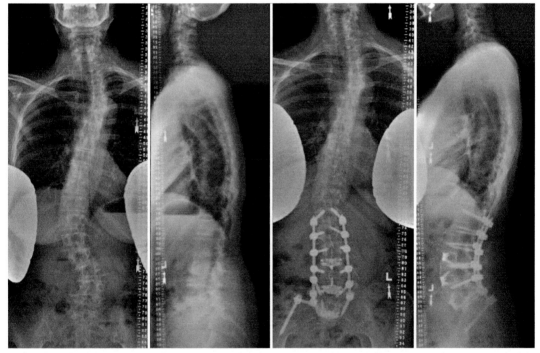

Fig. 13.4 Adult spinal deformity with imbalance successfully intervened by multilevel anterior lumbar interbody fusion and posterior instrumentation.

the superiority of one approach over another in terms of fusion or clinical outcomes. This is because there are minimal/no class I studies available to propose a definite LIF approach for a specific disease condition. Literature in LIF also lacks a strong comparison between approaches. Overall, MIS-TLIF results in a good fusion rate, better functional outcomes, less blood loss, and shorter ambulation and hospital stay in the management of DS. Furthermore, it is associated with less complication rates or resurgery. However, MIS techniques are costly and hence in limited resource setup, open TLIF should be the procedure of choice with better ODI scores compared with other open techniques. ALIF procedures achieve better postoperative DH and postoperative SL; however, PLIF has the greatest blood loss and does not have any advantage over the others in an ideal situation. Despite the type of approach, any surgery when meticulously done showed that postoperative outcomes and complication rates are similar across all approaches.

References

1. Mobbs RJ, Phan K, Malham G, Seex K, Rao PJ. Lumbar interbody fusion: techniques, indications and comparison of interbody fusion options including PLIF, TLIF, MI-TLIF, OLIF/ATP, LLIF and ALIF. J Spine Surg 2015;1(1):2–18

2. Hadra BE. Wiring of the spinous processes in Pott's disease. Trans Am Orthop Assoc. 1981;4:206

3. Harms JG, Jeszenszky D. Die posteriore, lumbale, interkorporelle Fusion in unilateraler transforaminaler Technik. Oper Orthop Traumatol 1998;10(2):90–102

4. de Kunder SL, Rijkers K, Caelers IJMH, de Bie RA, Koehler PJ, van Santbrink H. Lumbar interbody fusion: a historical overview and a future perspective. Spine 2018;43(16):1161–1168

5. Mobbs RJ, Phan K, Thayaparan GK, Rao PJ. Anterior lumbar interbody fusion as a salvage technique for pseudarthrosis following posterior lumbar fusion surgery. Global Spine J 2016;6(1):14–20

6. Koenig S, Jauregui JJ, Shasti M, et al. Decompression versus fusion for grade I degenerative spondylolisthesis: a meta-analysis. Global Spine J 2019;9(2):155–161

7. Chan AK, Bisson EF, Bydon M, et al. A comparison of minimally invasive transforaminal lumbar interbody fusion and decompression alone for degenerative lumbar spondylolisthesis. Neurosurg Focus 2019;46(5):E13

8. Xu DS, Walker CT, Godzik J, Turner JD, Smith W, Uribe JS. Minimally invasive anterior, lateral, and oblique lumbar interbody fusion: a literature review. Ann Transl Med 2018;6(6):104

9. Cho JY, Goh TS, Son SM, Kim DS, Lee JS. Comparison of anterior approach and posterior approach to instrumented interbody fusion for spondylolisthesis: a meta-analysis. World Neurosurg. 2019; pii: S1878–8750(19)31407-X

10. Teng I, Han J, Phan K, Mobbs R. A meta-analysis comparing ALIF, PLIF, TLIF and LLIF. J Clin Neurosci 2017;44:11–17

11. Keorochana G, Setrkraising K, Woratanarat P, Arirachakaran A, Kongtharvonskul J. Clinical outcomes after minimally invasive transforaminal lumbar interbody fusion and lateral lumbar interbody fusion for treatment of degenerative lumbar disease: a systematic review and meta-analysis. Neurosurg Rev 2018;41(3):755–770

12. Inamasu J, Guiot BH. Vascular injury and complication in neurosurgical spine surgery. Acta Neurochir (Wien) 2006;148(4):375–387

13. Brau SA, Delamarter RB, Schiffman ML, Williams LA, Watkins RG. Vascular injury during anterior lumbar surgery. Spine J 2004;4(4):409–412

14. Lindley EM, McBeth ZL, Henry SE, et al. Retrograde ejaculation after anterior lumbar spine surgery. Spine 2012;37(20):1785–1789

15. Sasso RC, Kenneth Burkus J, LeHuec JC. Retrograde ejaculation after anterior lumbar interbody fusion: transperitoneal versus retroperitoneal exposure. Spine 2003;28(10):1023–1026

16. Pichelmann MA, Dekutoski MB. Complications related to anterior and lateral lumbar surgery. Semin Spine Surg 2011;23(2):91–100

17. Hah R, Kang HP. Lateral and oblique lumbar interbody fusion-current concepts and a review of recent literature. Curr Rev Musculoskelet Med 2019. doi: 10.1007/s12178-019-09562-6. [Epub ahead of print]

18. Wu RH, Fraser JF, Härtl R. Minimal access versus open transforaminal lumbar interbody fusion: meta-analysis of fusion rates. Spine 2010;35(26): 2273–2281

19. Foley KT, Holly LT, Schwender JD. Minimally invasive lumbar fusion. Spine 2003;28(15, Suppl):S26–S35

20. Fujimori T, Le H, Schairer WW, Berven SH, Qamirani E, Hu SS. Does transforaminal lumbar interbody fusion have advantages over posterolateral lumbar fusion for degenerative spondylolisthesis? Global Spine J 2015;5(2): 102–109

21. Zhang Q, Yuan Z, Zhou M, Liu H, Xu Y, Ren Y. A comparison of posterior lumbar interbody fusion and transforaminal lumbar interbody fusion: a literature review and meta-analysis. BMC Musculoskelet Disord 2014;15:367

22. Lee JC, Kim Y, Soh JW, Shin BJ. Risk factors of adjacent segment disease requiring surgery after lumbar spinal fusion: comparison of posterior lumbar interbody fusion and posterolateral fusion. Spine 2014;39(5):E339–E345

23. Xie L, Wu WJ, Liang Y. Comparison between minimally invasive transforaminal lumbar interbody fusion and conventional open transforaminal lumbar interbody fusion: an updated meta-analysis. Chin Med J (Engl) 2016;129(16): 1969–1986

24. Qin R, Liu B, Zhou P, et al. Minimally invasive versus traditional open transforaminal lumbar interbody fusion for the treatment of single-level spondylolisthesis grades 1 and 2: a systematic review and meta-analysis. World Neurosurg 2019;122:180–189

25. Li A, Li X, Zhong Y. Is minimally invasive superior than open transforaminal lumbar interbody fusion for single-level degenerative lumbar diseases: a meta-analysis. J Orthop Surg Res 2018;13(1):241

26. Xie Q, Zhang J, Lu F, Wu H, Chen Z, Jian F. Minimally invasive versus open transforaminal lumbar interbody fusion in obese patients: a meta-analysis. BMC Musculoskelet Disord 2018; 19(1):15

27. Lin EY, Kuo YK, Kang YN. Effects of three common lumbar interbody fusion procedures for degenerative disc disease: a network meta-analysis of prospective studies. Int J Surg 2018; 60:224–230

Chapter 14
Intraoperative Neuromonitoring in Lumbar Interbody Fusion

14 Intraoperative Neuromonitoring in Lumbar Interbody Fusion

Dheeraj Masapu, Veeramani Preethish-Kumar

Introduction

Intraoperative neurophysiological monitoring (IONM) requires continuous evaluation of the central/peripheral nervous system during a surgical procedure when imminent injury is possible. IONM can either detect an iatrogenic injury allowing reversal or minimization of the injury and/or map critical structures during the procedure to avoid any damage. In lumbar interbody fusion (LIF), surgeons have always sought ways to minimize the inherent dangers of operating near the spinal cord and cauda equina nerve roots and plexus. Methods such as intraoperative and postoperative imaging have been used to confirm the proper placement of correction hardware, but many surgeons desire immediate feedback regarding patients' neurological status during surgery. Hence, usage of multimodal monitoring, such as somatosensory evoked potentials (SSEPs), motor evoked potentials (MEPs), and electromyograms (EMGs), triggered EMGs, enables proper monitoring of spinal cord and nerve roots in real time and also take measures to prevent or lessen irritation and potential damage. As evidenced by a large multicenter study, spinal surgeries that incorporate the feedback of an experienced neurophysiology team can have as much as a 50% lower rate of neurological deficits.[1] Successful use of this technology requires a coordinated three way communication between the neurosurgeon, neuroanesthesiologist, and neurophysiologist.

Methods of Evoked Potential Monitoring in Lumbar Spine Surgeries

The available methods for intraoperative neuromonitoring in lumbar spine surgeries are enumerated in **Box 14.1**.

Box 14.1 Methods for intraoperative neuromonitoring in lumbar spine surgeries

- Somatosensory evoked potentials
- Motor evoked potentials
- Triggered electromyogram
- Spontaneous electromyogram

Somatosensory Evoked Potentials

SSEPs are the most widely available and commonly used modality in spine surgery. They were initially described by Nash et al in 1977,[2] in which the distal stimulating electrodes are placed on the peripheral nerves of the limbs, and ascending sensory signals are recorded at the scalp, which corresponds to the somatosensory area of the cortex. The most common sites for stimulation are the posterior tibial for the lower extremities, and median nerve for the upper extremities.[3] SSEPs directly monitor the dorsal column-medial lemniscus pathway; however, they do not monitor the corticospinal pathways. Hence, care should be taken in suspected cases of focal corticospinal tract injury as in anterior spinal artery syndrome due to the potential chances of false negative results. Significant changes include a decrease in amplitude greater than 50% or an increase in latency more than 10% from baseline. Nuwer et al,[1] reported on the results of a multicenter survey of the members of Scoliosis Research Society. This survey yielded 51,263 cases in which SSEPs were used as the sole mode of neuromonitoring, with a sensitivity of 92% and a specificity of 98% in identifying new postoperative motor deficits (**Fig. 14.1a–d**).

Settings and Normative Data

- Current: 15 to 35 mA.
- Normal latency in median nerve: 20 ms (N20).

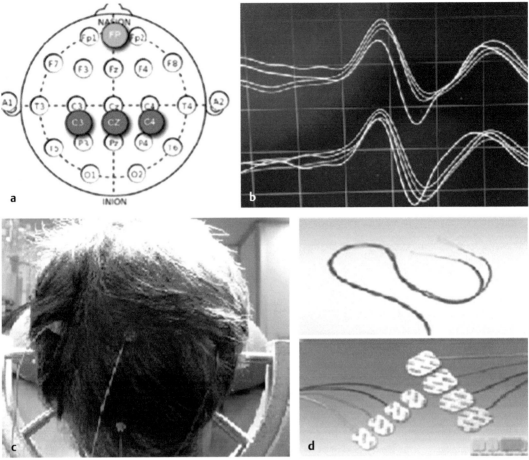

Fig. 14.1 (a) Placement of corkscrew electrodes on the scalp. **(b)** Somatosensory evoked potentials waves. **(c)** Corkscrew electrodes. **(d)** Needle electrodes and sticker electrodes for nerve stimulation.

- Normal latency in posterior tibial nerve: 37 ms (P37).

Motor Evoked Potentials

Merton and Morton in 1980,[4] described transcranial magnetic stimulation of the motor cortex, which made direct monitoring of the corticospinal pathway a possibility. This led to the development of transcranial MEPs monitoring during spinal surgery. The electrical stimulation is given at the C3 and C4 (scalp), which corresponds to the motor cortex of the brain. Multitrain stimuli can be used to overcome the effects of anesthesia and the signal passes through the corticospinal tract to evoke a response in the muscle called compound motor action potential (CMAP).

Interpretation of MEP Recording

Currently, four methods are routinely used for the interpretation of MEP responses:

(1) The all-or-none criterion, (2) the amplitude criterion, (3) the threshold criterion, and (4) the morphology criterion. The all-or-none criterion is the most widely cited and used method, given the inherent variability of signals in MEP monitoring.[5] Based on this approach, a complete loss of the MEP signal with previous preliminary baseline recording is indicative of a clinically significant event. A modification of the all-or-none approach involves measuring the CMAP amplitude at baseline, followed by the measurement of the relative change to determine if a clinically significant change has occurred.

Langeloo et al,[6] found a sensitivity of 100% in a series of 145 consecutive patients when monitored from six different sites, compared with a sensitivity of 88% when monitored at two sites only (**Fig. 14.2a–c**).

Settings

- Current used: 200 to 550 V.

- Train of stimuli: 4 to 8.

- Polarity of stimuli: normal, inverse, biphasic.

- Type of stimuli: single burst, double burst.

Triggered EMG Monitoring

Triggered EMG was initially described by Calancie et al[7] in a porcine model in 1992 as a means of assessing accuracy of pedicle screw placement. Triggered EMG relies on the concept that intact cortical bone should electrically insulate a well-placed pedicle screw from the adjacent nerve root. In contrast, the presence of medial pedicle and near nerve root breach, the pedicle screw would be relatively poorly insulated. Thus, by direct pedicle screw electrical stimulation and electromyographically assessing the lowest threshold voltage at

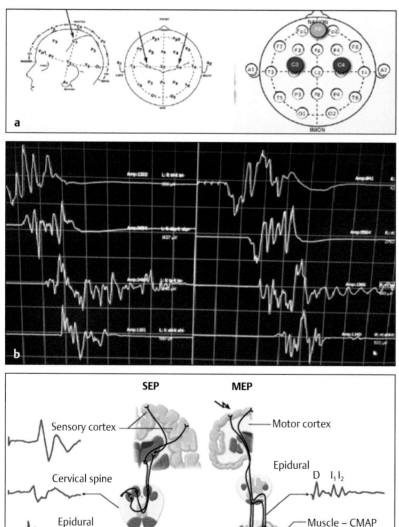

Fig. 14.2 (a) Electrode placement on scalp. **(b)** Compound motor action potentials from upper and lower limbs. **(c)** Somatosensory and motor evoked potential pathway.

which CMAPs are generated, one can assess the likelihood of medial pedicle breach. It is also very useful in detecting nerve root injuries. Triggered EMG has a particular utility in minimally invasive spine surgeries where visualization of the anatomical landmarks is limited. In such cases, stimulation of pedicle taps and K-wires may be used to evaluate accurate screw trajectory. Notably, in the setting of preoperative nerve root deficit, nerve conduction may be impaired, requiring higher thresholds for stimulation. In 2007, Raynor et al[8] reported the results of more than 4,800 consecutive lumbar pedicle screw placements, obtained by triggered EMG compared with postoperative CT scans. The authors found that with a threshold of more than 8.0 mA, there was a 99.5 to 99.8% likelihood of intraosseous screw placement. Based on the level of surgery, the muscles to be monitored will be decided and are based on the myotomal distribution (**Table 14.1**; **Fig. 14.3**).

Table 14.1 Innervation of different muscles of the lower limbs

Root	Muscle	Nerve
L-2, L-3	Iliacus	Lumbar plexus
L-3, L-4	Vastus lateralis, rectus femoris	Femoral nerve
L-4, L-5	Tibialis anterior	Peroneal nerve
L-5, S-1	Extensor hallucis longus	Peroneal
S-1, S-2	Abductor hallucis longus	Tibial
S2–S4	Striated urethral sphincter	Pudendal nerve
S-3, S-4, S-5	External anal sphincter	Pudendal nerve

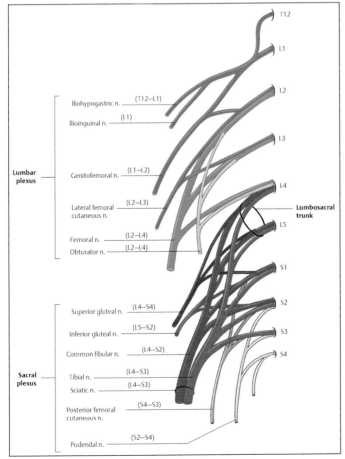

Fig. 14.3 The lumbosacral plexus. (Source: Lumbosacral Plexus. In: Socolovsky M, Rasulic L, Midha R et al., ed. Manual of Peripheral Nerve Surgery. From the Basics to Complex Procedures. 1st Edition. Thieme; 2017.)

Settings

- Electrode type: monopolar.
- Stimulus: 5 to 15 mA.

Spontaneous EMGs

Spontaneous or free-running EMG is widely used as a means of monitoring selective nerve root function during spinal cord surgery. No stimulation is required for this technique, and continuous recordings are made from pre-selected muscle groups based on the nerve roots at risk. At baseline, a healthy nerve root should show no muscle activity, that is, either a flat line or silence if audio feedback is equipped. During surgery, irritation of the nerve root due to traction or thermal injury will result in spikes or bursts of activity termed as neurotonic discharges (**Fig. 14.4**). Gunnarsson et al,[9] reported spontaneous EMG activation at least once in 77.5% of 213 consecutive lumbosacral cases, which resulted in a sensitivity of 100%, but a specificity of only 23.5%. Trains of higher frequency and/or amplitude tend to represent significant nerve fiber recruitment caused by

excessive force on the nerve and are likely to indicate a high probability of nerve injury if a relevant manipulation is sustained.

Anesthetic Concerns for Different Types of IONM

Motor Evoked Potentials

Muscle relaxants need to be avoided while monitoring MEPs including inhalational anesthetic agents, which has to be either avoided or used with a MAC of <0.5 to get good responses.[10] Total intravenous anesthesia with propofol will have the least effect on the MEP wave forms. Addition of adjuvants like dexmedetomidine and fentanyl to propofol will help in decreasing the dose of propofol required. Malcharek et al, compared the effects of desflurane and propofol on the MEP waveforms and found significant suppression of waves with desflurane.[11] Sloan et al, studied effects of addition of 3% minimum alveolar concentration (MAC) desflurane on the MEP waveforms and noticed that (3%)

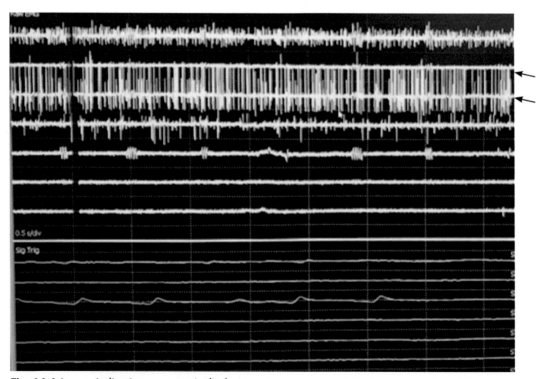

Fig. 14.4 Arrows indicating neurotonic discharges.

desflurane can be used in conjunction with SSEP and MEP monitoring for adult patients undergoing spine surgery.

Somatosensory Evoked Potentials

Somatosensory evoked potentials are sensitive to inhalational agents like sevoflurane and desflurane. The amplitude will decrease and latency will increase and the effects will be more pronounced when MAC is increased. Muscle relaxants can be used during the SSEP monitoring. Propofol has least effect on the SSEP wave forms.

EMGs (Spontaneous and Triggered)

Muscle relaxants need to be avoided during EMG monitoring as they will interfere with the recordings. Inhalational and intravenous anesthesia can be used during the maintenance of anesthesia. Opioids have minimal or no effect on the EMG recording (**Table 14.2**).

Multimodality Monitoring

The concept of multimodality monitoring relies on taking advantage of the individual strengths of its various submodalities, and is able to provide a more global and accurate assessment of the dorsal and ventral functions of the spinal cord. When EMG is added, the overall function of the nervous system can be monitored, from the level of cortex to the muscle. The combined use of SSEPs, MEPs, and both spontaneous and triggered EMG provides the necessary tools required to optimally monitor the functional integrity of the spinal cord during a broad spectrum of routine and complex spinal surgeries, while maximizing the diagnostic efficacy of monitoring in detecting neurological injury (**Table 14.3**).

Table 14.2 Effect of anesthesia on different modalities

Modality of monitoring	Inhalational anesthesia	Intravenous anesthesia	Muscle relaxants
MEP	Avoid or minimal use	Can be used	Avoid
SSEP	Avoid or minimal use	Can be used	Can be used
Triggered EMG	Can be used	Can be used	Avoid
Spontaneous EMG	Can be used	Can be used	Avoid

Abbreviations: EMG, electromyogram; MEP, motor evoked potentials; SSEP, somatosensory evoked potentials.

Table 14.3 Review of literature using multimodality monitoring in lumbar spine surgeries

Authors	Year	Total no. of cases	Deficits	sEMG	tEMG	SSEP	MEP
Darden et al[12]	1996	132	3		2(+)1(−)		
Welch et al[13]	1997	32	1	1(+)	1(+)		
Balzer et al[14]	1998	44	2	2(+)			
Bose et al[15]	2001	61	1	1(+)			
Iwasaki et al[16]	2003	817	2				2(−)
Macdonald et al[17]	2007	206	3				1(+) 2(−)
Santiago Pérez et al[18]	2007	54	1	1(−)	1(−)		
Lieberman man et al[19]	2008	35	10	6(+) 4(−)			10(+)
Alemo and Sayadipour[20]	2010	86	3	3(−)			
Raynor et al[8]	2013	12,375	4			4(+)	

Abbreviations: (+), positive signal changes; (−), negative signal changes; MEP, motor evoked potential; sEMG, spontaneous electromyography; SSEP, somatosensory evoked potential; tEMG, triggered electromyography.

Monitoring in Various Approaches of Lumbar Interbody Fusion

LIF is performed using five main approaches including posterior lumbar interbody fusion (PLIF), transforaminal lumbar interbody fusion (TLIF), oblique lumbar interbody fusion (OLIF), anterior lumbar interbody fusion (ALIF), and lateral lumbar interbody fusion (LLIF).

Monitoring Considerations in PLIF, TLIF

In the PLIF technique, surgical access to the intervertebral disc is from the posterior direction and hence there is a possibility of damaging the nerve roots during the procedure. This possibility of damaging the cauda equina and nerve roots is present, making the motor evoked potentials very useful during the surgery. In TLIF, the access is unilateral and hence nerve root monitoring (exiting/transverse) using triggered/spontaneous EMG is the main modality of monitoring. In the posterior approaches, roots are usually visualized and protected by dissecting the epidural fat and ligamentum flavum to get a clear window. Monitoring the exiting nerve root can salvage this step and prevent postoperative epidural fibrosis (**Fig. 14.5**). In a 2004 study, Gunnarsson et al[9] analyzed the sensitivity and specificity of detecting new postoperative motor deficits using multimodality monitoring during any thoracolumbar procedures. They reported that spontaneous electromyography has a sensitivity of 100% with a specificity of 23.7%. On the other hand, SSEPs provided a sensitivity of 28.6% with a specificity of 94.7%.

Monitoring Considerations in OLIF, LLIF

OLIF exploits a window between the prevertebral venous structures and anterior border of the psoas muscle to access the targeted disc. OLIF, unlike LLIF, might reduce the complications related to the lumbar plexus injury in the psoas muscle. In OLIF, monitoring is not as mandatory like direct lateral lumbar interbody fusion (DLIF) due to the lessened manipulation of psoas muscle and lumbar plexus. However, in DLIF, the neurophysiological intraoperative monitoring is mandatory to routinely monitor lumbar plexus during the surgery. Silvestre et al noted only a 3.9% rate of complication related to lumbar plexus injury or psoas muscle weakness following OLIF in 179 patients.[21] Another study done by Lee et al, assessing the utility of IONM in OLIF, has shown no difference in the postoperative outcomes between the IONM and non-IONM groups.[22]

Triggered EMG is the chief monitoring modality for the lumbar plexus but the placement of needles in the muscles is based on the motor supply of the lumbar plexus near the psoas muscle (**Table 14.4**; **Fig. 14.6**).

Monitoring Considerations in ALIF

ALIF is frequently performed and there are several potential mechanisms of lumbar nerve root injury during ALIF. For example, direct impact to the nerve roots can occur during graft insertion. In addition, pressure because of an expanding epidural hematoma can produce neurological deficits. Furthermore, the lumbosacral plexus is vulnerable during exposure and retraction. Reported rates of neurological

Table 14.4 Needle placement for EMG monitoring

Nerve/Muscle	Position of needle for EMG
Rectus femoris and/or vastus medialis (femoral nerve)	3–4 cm over the superior patellar edge
Gracilis (obturator nerve)	3–4 cm below the symphysis pubis
Lateral cutaneous femoral nerve	Immediately below the anterior superior iliac spine
Genitofemoral nerve	Cremaster (in men) or labium majus or femoral triangle (in women)
External oblique (Iliohypogastric/Ilioinguinal nerves)	Next to the linea semilunaris
Tibialis muscle (Lumbosacral trunk)	Lateral compartment of leg

Abbreviation: EMG, electromyogram.

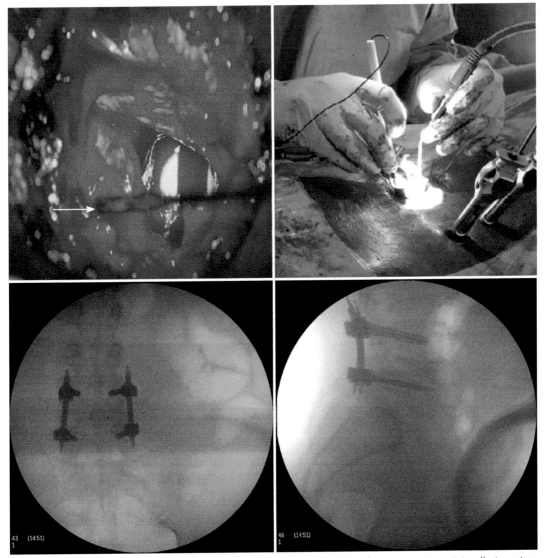

Fig. 14.5 Arrow showing the stimulator on exiting nerve root. Stimulator usage in minimally invasive-transforaminal lumbar interbody fusion and C-arm image after successful procedure.

deficit following ALIF range from 1 to 3%.[23] Exposures at L3/L4 and L2/L3 appeared less likely to results in positive alerts. This is probably because the retractors are deployed above the aortic bifurcation with less need for mobilizing the left iliac vessels than in most cases of L4/L5 exposure. Brau et al have previously demonstrated transient ischemia occurring in the lower extremities during ALIF at L4/L5 with the potential to reduce SSEP signals.[24] Although IONM technique involves monitoring only the posterior tibial nerve, neurological dysfunction due to vascular compromise would be expected to be detected irrespective of which peripheral nerve is monitored.[25]

Complications of IONM

The complications of IONM include pain or headache, kindling, accidental injury resulting from patient movement, tongue bite injuries, epidural complications, and disturbances of hormonal or hematological homeostasis.

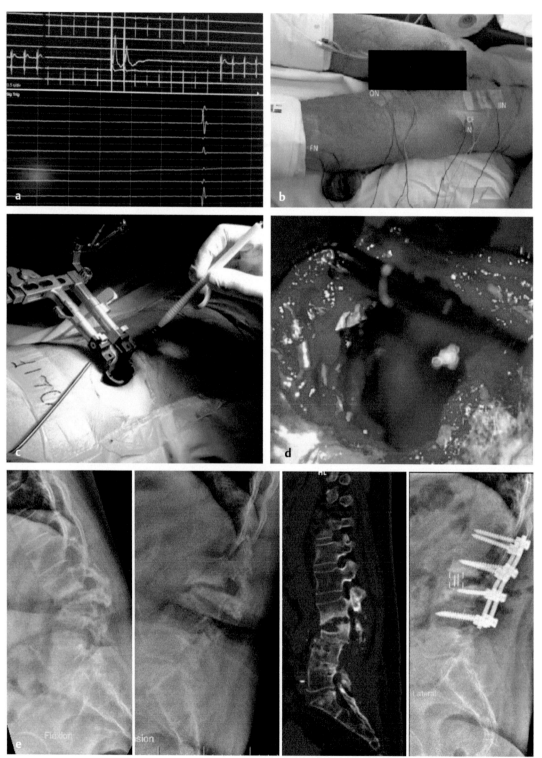

Fig. 14.6 (a) Triggered electromyogram. **(b)** Positioning of the registering electrodes according to lumbar plexus rami. **(c)** Usage of monopolar stimulator in the OLIF. **(d)** Stimulation of the surgical field. **(e)** Preoperative and postoperative X-ray, computed tomography images of the patient.

Very rare complications included are seizures, cognitive problems, cardiac arrhythmias, and scalp burns.

Tongue Bite

Cause: Strong temporalis muscle contraction with C3/4 stimulation. Jones et al reported one bitten tongue as a result of jaw muscle contraction during D185 pulse train transcranial electrical stimulation (TES) and advised bite blocks.[26] Calancie et al (2001) reported a unique mandibular fracture using C3/4 D185 stimulation in one patient without a bite block.[27] Prevention is by using bite block or more medial C12 stimulation.

Movement-Related Injury

The pulse trains and incomplete neuromuscular blockade can induce movement-related injuries or sometimes spontaneous activity also can cause injury. The strategies to decrease the increased movement are by adjusting stimulus intensity to minimal, partial neuromuscular blockade, preceding single-pulse TES by foot sole stimulation, or a priming tibialis anterior spinal motor neurons through the withdrawal reflex to respond to a single corticospinal volley.

Conclusion

IONM is a rapidly evolving field with the potential to greatly improve the safety of spinal surgery. A thorough appreciation of the strengths and weaknesses of each monitoring modality is critical for the optimal use of IONM. Preoperative discussion between the neurosurgeon, anesthesiologist, and electrophysiologist is an essential component of safe IONM usage, and topics should include anesthetic requirements for IONM, alarm criteria to be used, and steps to be taken in response to a positive alarm. Further prospective studies are needed to establish the true efficacy of IONM; but when used properly, IONM represents a powerful tool for improving outcomes in spine surgery. In a resourceful setup, IONM definitely compliments a surgeon in preventing the intraoperative complications as much as possible. However, a good anatomical knowledge is definitely the main criterion for any type of surgery and its success even when these highly advanced infrastructures are not available.

References

1. Nuwer MR, Dawson EG, Carlson LG, Kanim LE, Sherman JE. Somatosensory evoked potential spinal cord monitoring reduces neurologic deficits after scoliosis surgery: results of a large multicenter survey. Electroencephalogr Clin Neurophysiol 1995;96(1):6–11

2. Nash CL Jr, Lorig RA, Schatzinger LA, Brown RH. Spinal cord monitoring during operative treatment of the spine. Clin Orthop Relat Res 1977; (126):100–105

3. May DM, Jones SJ, Crockard HA. Somatosensory evoked potential monitoring in cervical surgery: identification of pre- and intraoperative risk factors associated with neurological deterioration. J Neurosurg 1996;85(4):566–573

4. Merton PA, Morton HB. Stimulation of the cerebral cortex in the intact human subject. Nature 1980;285(5762):227

5. Kothbauer KF, Deletis V, Epstein FJ. Motor-evoked potential monitoring for intramedullary spinal cord tumor surgery: correlation of clinical and neurophysiological data in a series of 100 consecutive procedures. Neurosurg Focus 1998; 4(5):e1

6. Langeloo DD, Lelivelt A, Louis Journée H, Slappendel R, de Kleuver M. Transcranial electrical motor-evoked potential monitoring during surgery for spinal deformity: a study of 145 patients. Spine 2003;28(10):1043–1050

7. Calancie B, Lebwohl N, Madsen P, Klose KJ. Intraoperative evoked EMG monitoring in an animal model. A new technique for evaluating pedicle screw placement. Spine 1992;17(10): 1229–1235

8. Raynor BL, Lenke LG, Bridwell KH, Taylor BA, Padberg AM. Correlation between low triggered electromyographic thresholds and lumbar pedicle screw malposition: analysis of 4857 screws. Spine 2007;32(24):2673–2678

9. Gunnarsson T, Krassioukov AV, Sarjeant R, Fehlings MG. Real-time continuous intraoperative electromyographic and somatosensory evoked potential recordings in spinal surgery: correlation of clinical and electrophysiologic findings in a prospective, consecutive series of 213 cases. Spine 2004;29(6):677–684

10. Macdonald DB. Intraoperative motor evoked potential monitoring: overview and update. J Clin Monit Comput 2006;20(5):347–377

11. Malcharek MJ, Loeffler S, Schiefer D, et al. Transcranial motor evoked potentials during

anesthesia with desflurane versus propofol—a prospective randomized trial. Clin Neurophysiol 2015;126(9):1825–1832

12. Darden BV II, Wood KE, Hatley MK, Owen JH, Kostuik J. Evaluation of pedicle screw insertion monitored by intraoperative evoked electromyography. J Spinal Disord 1996;9(1):8–16

13. Welch WC, Rose RD, Balzer JR, Jacobs GB. Evaluation with evoked and spontaneous electromyography during lumbar instrumentation: a prospective study. J Neurosurg 1997;87(3):397–402

14. Balzer JR, Rose RD, Welch WC, Sclabassi RJ. Simultaneous somatosensory evoked potential and electromyographic recordings during lumbosacral decompression and instrumentation. Neurosurgery 1998;42(6):1318–1324, discussion 1324–1325

15. Bose B, Wierzbowski LR, Sestokas AK. Neurophysiologic monitoring of spinal nerve root function during instrumented posterior lumbar spine surgery. Spine 2002;27(13):1444–1450

16. Iwasaki H, Tamaki T, Yoshida M, et al. Efficacy and limitations of current methods of intraoperative spinal cord monitoring. J Orthop Sci 2003;8(5):635–642

17. Macdonald DB, Stigsby B, Al Homoud I, Abalkhail T, Mokeem A. Utility of motor evoked potentials for intraoperative nerve root monitoring. J Clin Neurophysiol 2012;29(2):118–125

18. Santiago-Pérez S, Nevado-Estévez R, Aguirre-Arribas J, Pérez-Conde MC. Neurophysiological monitoring of lumbosacral spinal roots during spinal surgery: continuous intraoperative electromyography (EMG). Electromyogr Clin Neurophysiol 2007;47(7-8):361–367

19. Lieberman JA, Lyon R, Feiner J, Hu SS, Berven SH. The efficacy of motor evoked potentials in fixed sagittal imbalance deformity correction surgery. Spine 2008;33(13):E414–E424

20. Alemo S, Sayadipour A. Role of intraoperative neurophysiologic monitoring in lumbosacral spine fusion and instrumentation: a retrospective study. World Neurosurg 2010;73(1):72–76, discussion e7

21. Silvestre C, Mac-Thiong J-M, Hilmi R, Roussouly P. Complications and morbidities of mini-open anterior retroperitoneal lumbar interbody fusion: oblique lumbar interbody fusion in 179 patients. Asian Spine J 2012;6(2):89–97

22. Lee HJ, Ryu KS, Hur JW, Seong JH, Cho HJ, Kim JS. Safety of lateral interbody fusion surgery without intraoperative monitoring. Turk Neurosurg 2018; 28(3):428–433

23. Bendersky M, Solá C, Muntadas J, et al. Monitoring lumbar plexus integrity in extreme lateral transpsoas approaches to the lumbar spine: a new protocol with anatomical bases. Eur Spine J 2015;24(5):1051–1057

24. Brau SA, Spoonamore MJ, Snyder L, et al. Nerve monitoring changes related to iliac artery compression during anterior lumbar spine surgery. Spine J 2003;3(5):351–355

25. Nuwer MR. Intraoperative monitoring of the spinal cord. Clin Neurophysiol 2008;119(2):247

26. Jones SJ, Harrison R, Koh KF, Mendoza N, Crockard HA. Motor evoked potential monitoring during spinal surgery: responses of distal limb muscles to transcranial cortical stimulation with pulse trains. Electroencephalogr Clin Neurophysiol 1996;100(5):375–383

27. Calancie B, Harris W, Broton JG, Alexeeva N, Green BA. "Threshold-level" multipulse transcranial electrical stimulation of motor cortex for intraoperative monitoring of spinal motor tracts: description of method and comparison to somatosensory evoked potential monitoring. J Neurosurg 1998;88(3):457–470

Chapter 15
Case Vignettes

- ➢ Case 1
  - Procedure of Choice—TLIF
- ➢ Case 2
  - Procedure of Choice—MIS TLIF
- ➢ Case 3
  - Procedure of Choice—OLIF with Percutaneous Pedicle Screw Fixation
- ➢ Case 4
  - Procedure of Choice—ALIF with Pedicle Screw Instrumentation
- ➢ Case 5
  - Procedure of Choice—OLIF

15 Case Vignettes

Case 1

A 68-year-old obese lady presented with difficulty in walking beyond 100 m for last 1 year. She also complained of low back ache (visual analog scale [VAS]-7) with bilateral leg pain (VAS 8; right > left L4 dermatome). She had neurogenic claudication and significant restriction in activities of daily living. She was hypertensive and had a previous history of retroperitoneal renal surgery. On examination she had bilateral ankle dorsiflexion (⅗) and extensor hallucis longus (EHL-3+) weakness on right side.

X-ray revealed osteoporosis and anterolisthesis at L3–4 and retrolisthesis at L4–5 with dynamic mobility (**Fig. 15.1a–c**).

Whole spine radiograph (**Fig. 15.2**) demonstrates an evolving degenerative lumbar scoliosis with C7 plumb line falling 4 cm in front of S1, and reduced lumbar lordosis.

MRI (**Fig. 15.3a–c**) shows significant canal stenosis at L3–4 with extruded disc and L4–5 canal stenosis secondary to facet hypertrophy, ligamentum flavum hypertrophy with modic changes.

She underwent open transforaminal lumbar interbody fusion (TLIF) procedure at L3–4, L4–5 with adequate decompression of L2–3, L3–4, and L4–5 levels. Postoperatively, she had improvement in her leg pain and walking distance. The whole spine radiograph (**Fig. 15.4a and b**) revealed C7 plumb line corrected by 2 cm in front of S1 and reasonably balanced alignment.

Procedure of Choice—TLIF

- Neurological deficits including urinary incontinence more than back pain: require adequate bilateral and wide decompression, which is better in open procedures.

- History of retroperitoneal surgery: chances of retroperitoneal scarring preclude anterior procedure.

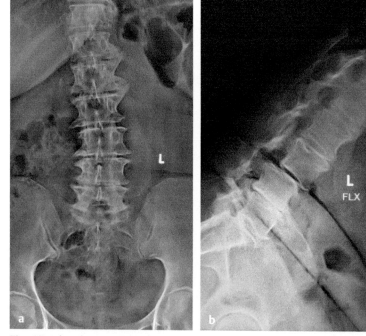
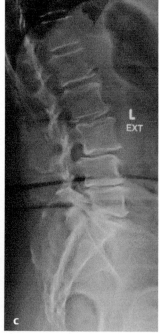

Fig. 15.1 (a–c) Dynamic radiograph demonstrating instability at L3–4 and L4–L5.

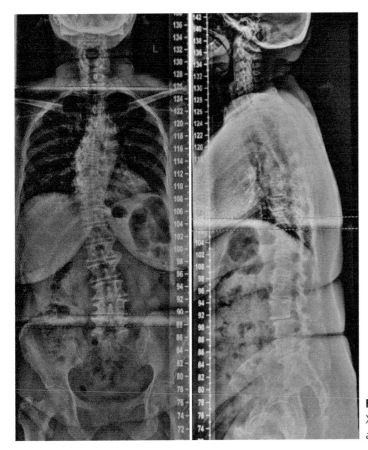

Fig. 15.2 Whole spine standing X-ray revealing sagittal and coronal abnormality.

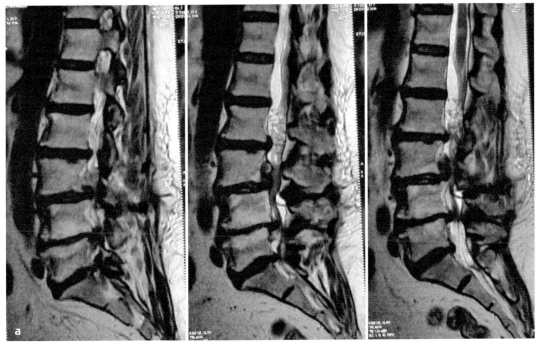

Fig. 15.3 (a) Magnetic resonance imaging demonstrating significant canal stenosis from L2–L5 with cranially migrated L3–L4 extruded disc *(Continued)*.

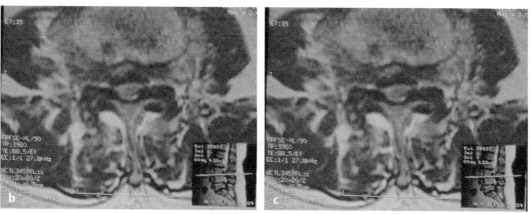

Fig. 15.3 *(Continued)* **(b and c)** Magnetic resonance imaging demonstrating significant canal stenosis from L2–L5 with cranially migrated L3–L4 extruded disc.

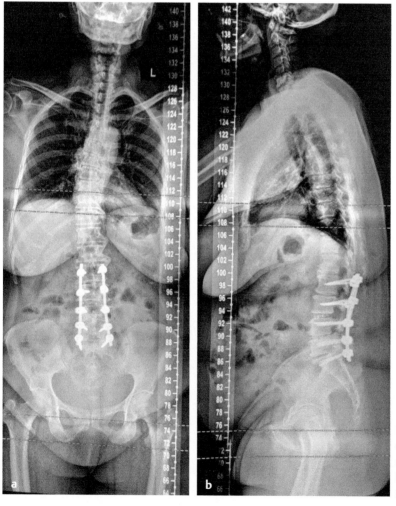

Fig. 15.4 (a and b) Postoperative whole spine standing X-ray with L2–S1 instrumentation with satisfactory balance.

Case 2

A 45-year-old male came with complaints of leg pain (VAS-8) of 1-month duration along L5 dermatome. He had similar complaints in the past but of less severity. He also had back pain at rest (VAS 5) which gets aggravated on bending forward (VAS 7). He had numbness along the lateral aspect of the leg. Examination revealed EHL weakness (⅗) and poor activities of daily living. SF-36 had poor physical composite score (PCS) (40%) and mental composite score (MCS) was 60%. His radiographs (**Fig. 15.5a–c**) showed a mobile degenerative grade I L4–5 spondylolisthesis. He underwent an MRI (**Fig 15.6a and b**) that revealed him to have L4–5 disc prolapse and facet arthritis compromising the spinal canal and lateral recess.

Minimally invasive surgery transforaminal lumbar interbody fusion (MIS TLIF) was performed on the left side. A large extruded disc was removed through left-sided facetectomy

and bean cage of 10 mm × 24 mm was inserted. Postoperatively, he had significant relief in leg pain and improvement in Roland-Morris back pain questionnaire by 70%. His SF-36 improved to PCS-60% and MCS-70%, respectively. His follow-up at 6 months showed good consolidation of graft with Bridwell grade II fusion (**Fig. 15.7**).

Procedure of Choice—MIS TLIF

- Back pain: MIS results in less muscle damage and chances of iatrogenic muscle fibrosis are reduced.

- Radiculopathy: secondary to disc prolapse and lateral recess stenosis with compression on traversing root which needs direct decompression. In addition, the disc height is preserved with no foraminal narrowing.

- Minimal blood loss and early recovery with equal fusion compared with open procedure.

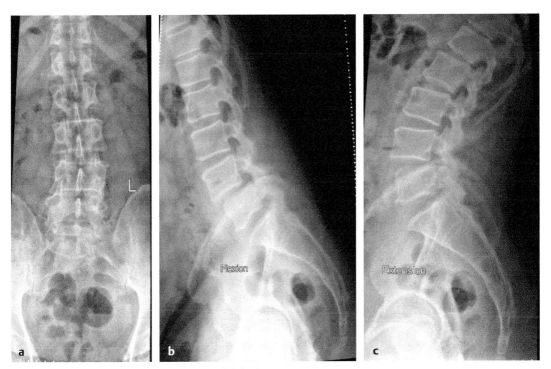

Fig. 15.5 (a–c) X-ray showing L4–L5 spondylolisthesis.

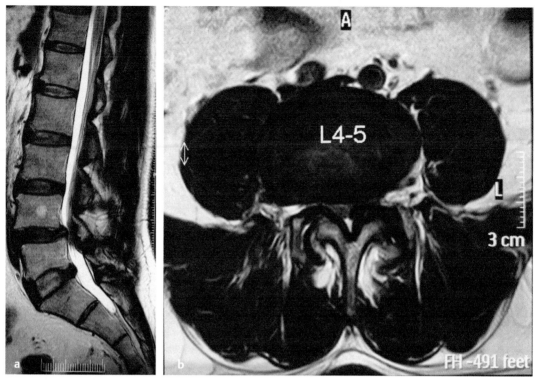

Fig. 15.6 (a and b) L4–L5 disc prolapse with nerve root compression on the left side.

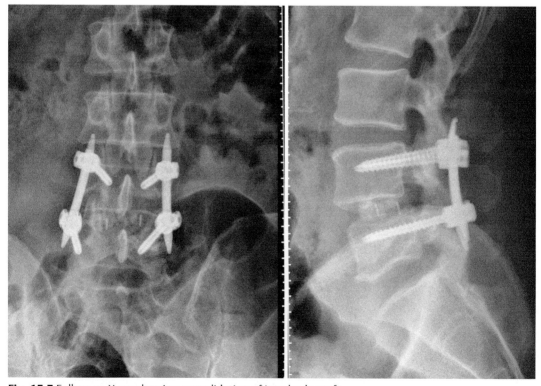

Fig. 15.7 Follow-up X-ray showing consolidation of interbody graft.

Case 3

A 70-year-old female was suffering from low back ache and mild numbness in the left leg for 6 years. The symptoms were tolerable. However, in the recent year, low back pain was getting worse. Meanwhile, she was not able to stand for long because of the trunk inclination to the front and right. She is a known case of ischemic heart disease and is also a diabetic. X-ray (standing and bending) showed that it

was a rigid and stiff deformity (**Fig. 15.8a–d**). It was refractory to conservative treatment. The patient was admitted to the hospital.

Considering patient's age and the morbidity of open correction surgery, she was supposed to be operated by a staged MIS surgery. The whole spine standing films were carefully analyzed (**Fig. 15.9**)

A stable, balanced spine was achieved with stage 1 oblique lateral interbody fusion (OLIF) surgery. The disc space manipulation was done

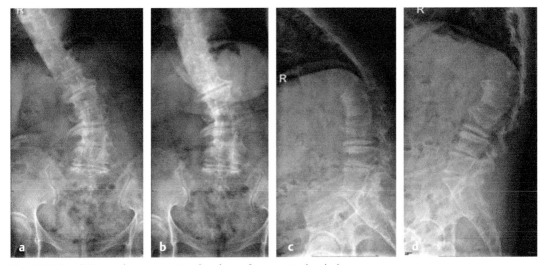

Fig. 15.8 (a–d) X-ray demonstrating fixed significant spinal imbalance.

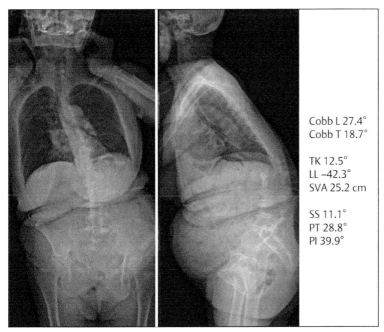

Cobb L 27.4°
Cobb T 18.7°

TK 12.5°
LL –42.3°
SVA 25.2 cm

SS 11.1°
PT 28.8°
PI 39.9°

Fig. 15.9 Whole spine X-ray showing pelvis parameter values, including sagittal and coronal values.

sequentially from L4/5 to L1/2 by means of annulotomy and end plate preparation. Prompt cages impacted with allograft were then inserted by slight knocking (**Fig. 15.10**).

The patient was mobilized the next day and follow-up X-ray films showed that her spinal deformity has been tremendously corrected not only coronally but also sagittally (**Fig. 15.11**).

One week after initial surgery, she underwent percutaneous pedicle screw implantation to secure the correction and spine balance. Patient had 2 years postoperative follow-up with complete satisfaction although there was a mild proximal junctional kyphosis on the standing films (**Fig. 15.12**).

Procedure of Choice—OLIF with Percutaneous Pedicle Screw Fixation

- Sagittal and coronal imbalance secondary to disc degenerations: multiple level anterior procedure (OLIF) increases disc height symmetrically, corrects the coronal and sagittal deformities.

- Back pain with significant disability: MIS percutaneous pedicle screw fixation limits muscle damage.

- Older age with co-morbidities: MIS has reduced blood loss and early postoperative recovery.

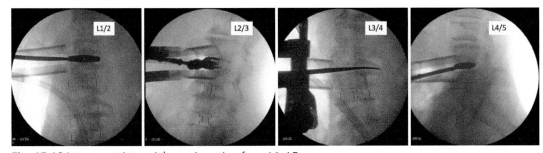

Fig. 15.10 Intraoperative serial cage insertion from L1–L5.

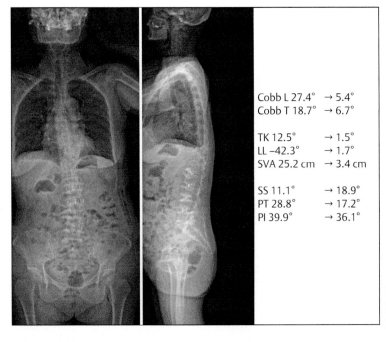

Cobb L 27.4° → 5.4°
Cobb T 18.7° → 6.7°

TK 12.5° → 1.5°
LL −42.3° → 1.7°
SVA 25.2 cm → 3.4 cm

SS 11.1° → 18.9°
PT 28.8° → 17.2°
PI 39.9° → 36.1°

Fig. 15.11 Immediate stage 1 postoperative X-ray showing proper alignment of the spine.

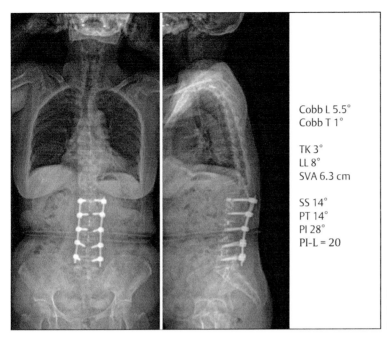

Cobb L 5.5°
Cobb T 1°

TK 3°
LL 8°
SVA 6.3 cm

SS 14°
PT 14°
PI 28°
PI-L = 20

Fig. 15.12 A 2-year follow-up X-ray with maintained correction.

Case 4

A 77-year-old female presented with low back ache and bilateral leg pain of a long duration. She was resistant to conservative management. Preoperative posteroanterior (PA) and lateral radiographs showed thoracolumbar scoliosis and stenosis from severe lumbar spondylosis **(Fig. 15.13)**.

She received an L2-S1 anterior lumbar interbody fusion (ALIF) and MIS L1-pelvis posterior spinal instrumented fusion **(Fig. 15.14)**

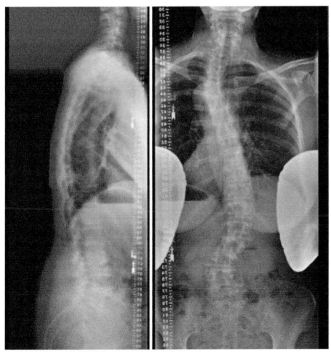

Fig. 15.13 Posteroanterior radiographs demonstrating degenerative scoliosis.

Postoperative (right) PA radiographs showed excellent correction of the deformity (**Fig. 15.15**).

Procedure of Choice—ALIF with Pedicle Screw Instrumentation

- Adult spinal deformity with sagittal and coronal imbalance: multiple level anterior procedure (ALIF—mainly to restore L5–S1 lordosis) corrects the deformity and maintains the spinal balance.

- Posterior pedicle screw fixation with right iliac screw fixation: left-sided lumbar scoliosis and to maintain lumbar lordosis.

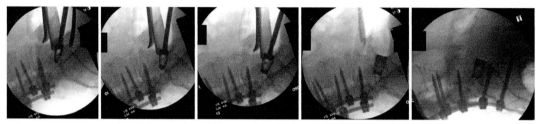

Fig. 15.14 Intraoperative fluoroscopy showing serial anterior lumbar interbody fusion cage placement.

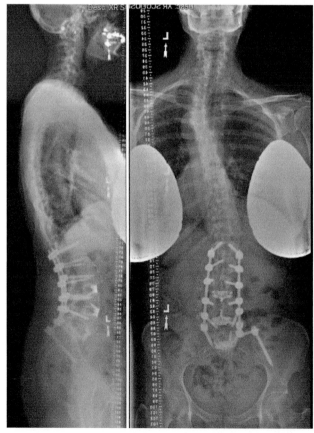

Fig. 15.15 Postoperative posteroanterior X-ray revealing excellent correction.

Case 5

A 59-year-old male came with a low back pain (VAS 7) for more than 5 years duration. He was not able to maintain upright posture or walk for long time followed by L4 radiculopathy. His Oswestry Disability Index (ODI) score was 70%. These symptoms were refractory to conservative treatment such as nonsteroidal anti-inflammatory drugs, physiotherapy, acupuncture, and traditional medicine. He was diagnosed with isthmic spondylolisthesis and collapsed disc space at L4–L5 level (**Fig. 15.16a–d**).

He underwent OLIF procedure with 10 mm × 50 mm-long cage and posterior percutaneous pedicle screw fixation in the same sitting. C-arm and postoperative X-ray films showed that the disc space was enlarged and the sagittal alignment was tremendously improved (**Fig. 15.17**).

He improved significantly in back pain and was relieved from radicular symptoms . His ODI score reduced to 10% and he became socially active.

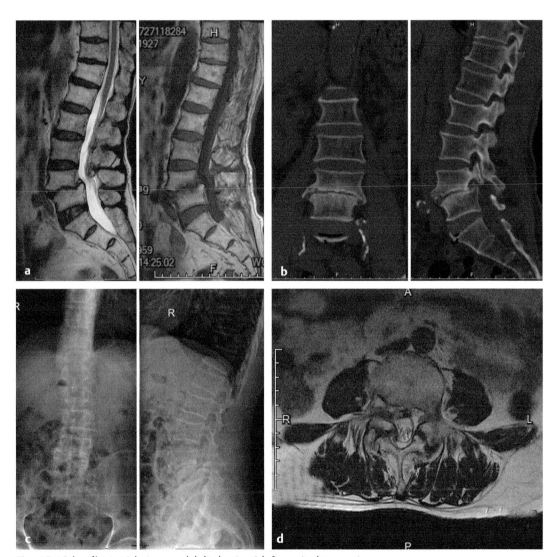

Fig. 15.16 (a–d) L4–L5 lytic spondylolisthesis with foraminal narrowing.

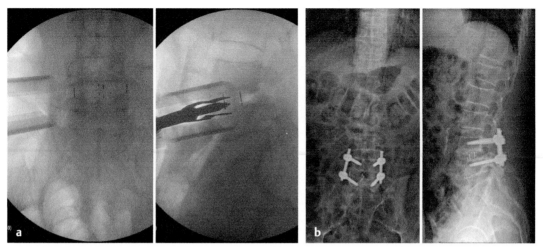

Fig. 15.17 Intraoperative oblique lateral interbody fusion cage placement **(a)** and postoperative radiograph with implants in proper position **(b)**.

Procedure of Choice—OLIF

- Back pain more than leg pain: good fusion is better with anterior procedures (e.g., OLIF) as it has good disc clearance and end plate preparation.

- Collapsed disc space with exiting nerve-related radiculopathy needs foraminal height restoration.

- Percutaneous pedicle screw fixation reduces slippage with minimal blood loss and muscle damage.

Index